Acute Psychiatric Emergencies

SECOND EDITION

Acute Psychiatric Emergencies

A Practical Approach

SECOND EDITION

Advanced Life Support Group

EDITED BY

Mark Buchanan
Consultant in Adult and Paediatric Emergency Medicine,
Arrowe Park Hospital,
Wirral University Teaching Hospital NHS Trust;
Honorary Clinical Senior Lecturer,
University of Liverpool

Damien Longson
Consultant Liaison Psychiatrist,
Greater Manchester Mental Health NHS Foundation Trust;
Honorary Professor of Psychiatry,
University of Manchester

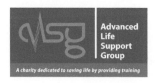

WILEY

Registered Offices
John Wiley & Sons, Inc., 111 River Street, Hoboken, NJ 07030, USA
John Wiley & Sons Ltd, New Era House, 8 Oldlands Way, Bognor Regis, West Sussex, PO22 9NQ

For details of our global editorial offices, customer services, and more information about Wiley products visit us at www.wiley.com.

The manufacturer's authorized representative according to the EU General Product Safety Regulation is Wiley-VCH GmbH, Boschstr. 12, 69469 Weinheim, Germany, e-mail: Product_Safety@wiley.com.

Wiley also publishes its books in a variety of electronic formats and by print-on-demand. Some content that appears in standard print versions of this book may not be available in other formats.

Library of Congress Cataloging-in-Publication Data Applied for:

Paperback ISBN: 9781394286263

Cover Design: Wiley
Cover Image: Courtesy of Sinead Kay, © fizkes/Getty Images, © Jacob Wackerhausen/Getty Images

Set in 9.5/11.5pt Montserrat by Straive, Pondicherry, India
Printed and bound by CPI Group (UK) Ltd, Croydon, CR0 4YY

C9781394286263_150325

Note to text:

Drugs and their doses are mentioned in this text. Although every effort has been made to ensure accuracy, the writers, editors, publishers and printers cannot accept liability for errors or omissions. The final responsibility for delivery of the correct dose remains with the physician prescribing and administering the drug.

Dedication

We would like to acknowledge and dedicate this manual to ALSG's former Chair of Trustees (1990–2024), Professor Kevin Mackway-Jones, in bringing the Acute Psychiatric Emergencies (APEx) course to fruition. By bringing together colleagues from across the acute and mental healthcare sectors, his vision, inspiration and beliefs turned the thought-provoking idea of essential mental health training that covers emergency management, wherever the setting, into reality.

Contents

Contributors to second edition

Roger Alcock MBChB, BSc(Hons), FRCP Edin, DCH, FRCEM, FRGS, Consultant in Emergency Medicine and Paediatric Emergency Medicine, Victoria Hospital, NHS Fife

Sally Arnold MBChB, MRCPsych, DRCOG, MA. Consultant Perinatal Psychiatrist, Midlands Partnership NHS Foundation Trust

Mark Buchanan FCEM, Consultant in Adult and Paediatric Emergency Medicine, Arrowe Park Hospital, Wirral University Teaching Hospital NHS Trust; Honorary Clinical Senior Lecturer, University of Liverpool

Rebecca Chubb MRCPsych, Locum Consultant Psychiatrist, North Staffordshire Combined Healthcare NHS Trust

Alys Cole-King MB, BCh, DGM, MSc, FRCPsych, Clinical Director, 4 Mental Health/retired Consultant Liaison Psychiatrist

Sandrine Dénéréaz Paramedic, Master in Public Administration, Paramedic School Director, Lausanne, Switzerland

James Ferguson FRCSEd, FRCS(A&E), FRCEM, FRCPE, FRSM, Consultant Surgeon in Emergency Medicine, NHS Grampian

Damien Longson PhD, FRCPsych, Consultant Liaison Psychiatrist, Greater Manchester Mental Health NHS Foundation Trust; Honorary Professor of Psychiatry, University of Manchester

Aaron McMeekin MBChB, LLB(Hons), MSc(Oxon), MRCPsych, PGCertMedEd, FHEA, Consultant Perinatal Psychiatrist, Greater Manchester Mental Health NHS Foundation Trust; Honorary Senior Clinical Teacher, Academic Unit of Medical Education, University of Sheffield

Andrew M. Russell MBChB, MRCS, FRCEM, Consultant in Emergency Medicine, University Hospital Monklands, Lanarkshire

Murray Smith MRCPsych, Consultant Liaison Psychiatrist, Department of Psychological Medicine, Aberdeen Royal Infirmary, NHS Grampian

Preface to second edition

The prevalence of mental health distress is increasing and is thought to account for up to 5% of presentations to Emergency Departments (EDs) in England. In 2023–24 there were over 200 000 ED attendances in England where the chief complaint could be identified as a definite or possible mental health issues. The two main reasons for presentation were suicidal thoughts or self-injurious behaviours. Other diagnoses included depression, anxiety, psychotic disorders and, although not necessarily mental health-related, substance misuse disorders.

In August 2024 there were 31 328 new referrals to psychiatric liaison teams in ED. Distress associated with the emergency situation is compounded by additional factors. For example, in the same time period more than 80 000 people experiencing a mental health crisis waited in an ED for more than 12 hours with 26 000 spending more than 24 hours in that setting.

Mental health emergencies present in many settings: prehospital in the patient's home or in the community, out-patient departments, emergency departments, acute wards and mental health wards; the response to patients in crisis is best seen as being multiagency: including general practitioners, ED staff, psychiatrist trained staff, paramedics, police and social services to name a few.

The new edition of the Acute Psychiatric Emergencies (APEx) course builds on our experience of running the course in several nations for the past 5 years. We wanted to strengthen the collaborative approach, review acronyms, update key principles and include emerging concepts of pivotal importance in supporting a patient in crisis. This book, with its 2-day hands on experiential course has been designed to bring teams together to work towards providing safe effective care to patients presenting with acute mental health symptoms in any setting. In the spirit of the collaboration taught on the course, the revised course and book has been completely revised by emergency and psychiatric physicians experienced in dealing with mental health emergencies.

The fundamental principles of the course have not changed. APEx is a structured, flexible and systematic approach for staff supporting patients in mental health crisis, whatever the setting. The APEx approach facilitates safe effective management and promotes joint, parallel working between specialities.

As before, APEx considers both mental and non-mental health-related behavioural disturbances with topics varying from organic presentations, de-escalation and mental health assessments. Into this second edition we have added sections on specific circumstances such as eating disorder emergencies and safety plans. We have introduced important new tools such as the SMART screening tool for triage, and refined the mental state acronyms to improve communication between acute and mental health specialities. The section on human factors has been updated and as always the course places the patient experience and patient safety at the heart of the clinical pathway.

Patients in a mental health crisis deserve better care. A caring, systematic and communicating approach is the start to making this happen.

Mark Buchanan and Damien Longson
January 2025

Preface to first edition

Emergency departments offer open access healthcare 24 hours a day, 7 days a week, 365 days a year. The number of patients attending these departments in England increased by 7.4% between 2010–11 and 2016–17 and is currently at an all-time high. It is unsurprising that a significant proportion of the patients attending emergency departments present with mental health problems, and the number of patients in crisis is increasing at 10% per year and now make up more than 5% (one in 20) of all attenders.

Despite the high numbers of patients attending in mental health crisis (more attend with this presentation than attend with chest pain), the vast majority of emergency department staff are not trained specifically to deal with patients with mental health emergencies or, indeed, to deal with mental illness at all. A value clarification exercise that looked into emergency mental healthcare in one emergency department in London established that the work most valued by the staff was trauma 'because of the excitement and drama it provided'. The environmental values for good mental healthcare (privacy, quietness, safety, calmness and having time) were noted to be the 'antithesis' of the environment found in the emergency department. Experienced emergency department nurses noted a 'deficit in mental health knowledge' but were unable to further identify the deficits. A key theme emerged of 'a perceived conflict between two cultures' which gives mental health a low status.

The course that this book supports (APEx) is designed to fill some of the gap and more closely align the cultures of care. The content has been designed jointly by psychiatrists and emergency physicians and is presented in a structured manner. Recognisable presentations (such as 'overdose and poisoning', 'aggression' and 'behaving strangely') are dealt with rather than focusing on diagnoses. Primary assessment is achieved with a new bespoke structured approach (ABCD AEIO U) that is similar to the more familiar ABCD emergency care approach to physical emergencies. Secondary assessment consists of parallel physical and psychosocial history and examinations. Throughout the text close co-operation between emergency and mental health teams is emphasised as is the value of joint working.

Patients in mental health crisis clearly deserve better than they currently get. This book, and the APEx course it supports, is for them.

Kevin Mackway-Jones
Manchester 2019

Acknowledgments

A great many people have put a lot of hard work into the production of this book, and the accompanying Acute Psychiatric Emergencies course. The Editors would like to thank all the contributors for their efforts.

We are greatly indebted to Kirsten Baxter, Kate Denning and Kelly Flaherty for their exceptional hard work and dedication towards this publication; their encouragement and guidance throughout the process has been gratefully received.

We would like to express our special thanks to Dr Alys Cole-King, Clinical Director at 4 Mental Health, for the Safety Planning section and use of the Safety Plan template.

Thanks to Catherine Giaquinto for designing the new algorithms and artwork for this edition.

Thanks to Chloe Cobb for her work with the SMART tool.

For the shared use of their images, resources and algorithms, we would like to thank:

eMentalHealth.ca - ASEPTIC Mental Status Examination (MSE) resource
Henry Murray, Pharmacist
Manchester Triage Group
SMART Form, Sierra Sacramento Valley Medical Society

We acknowledge the contribution of Satveer Nijjar, Independent Trainer with Lived Experience, 'Attention Seekers Training', who provided her personal account to inform Chapter 14 'The patient experience'.

Contact details and website information

ALSG: www.alsg.org

For details on ALSG courses visit the website or contact:

Advanced Life Support Group
ALSG Centre for Training and Development
29–31 Ellesmere Street
Swinton, Manchester
M27 0LA
Tel: +44 (0) 161 794 1999
Email: enquiries@alsg.org

Updates

The material contained within this book is updated on approximately a 4-yearly cycle. However, practice may change in the interim period. We will post any changes on the ALSG website, so we advise you to visit the website regularly to check for updates (www.alsg.org).

On-line feedback

It is important to ALSG that the contact with our providers continues after a course is completed. We now contact everyone 6 months after their course has taken place asking for on-line feedback on the course. This information is then used whenever the course is updated to ensure that the course provides optimum training to its participants.

How to use your textbook

The anytime, anywhere textbook

Wiley E-Text

Your textbook comes with free access to a **Wiley E-Text: Powered by VitalSource** version – a digital version of this textbook which you own as soon as you download it.

Your **Wiley E-Text** allows you to:

Search: Save time by finding terms and topics instantly in your book, your notes, even your whole library (once you've downloaded more textbooks)

Note and highlight: Colour code, highlight and make digital notes right in the text so you can find them quickly and easily

Organize: Keep books, notes and class materials organized in folders inside the application

Share: Exchange notes and highlights with others

Upgrade: Your textbook can be transferred when you need to change or upgrade computers

The **Wiley E-Text** version will also allow you to copy and paste any photograph or illustration into assignments, presentations and your own notes.

To access your Wiley E-Text:

- Find the redemption code on the inside front cover of this book and carefully scratch away the top coating of the label. Visit **http://www.vitalsource.com/downloads** to download the Bookshelf application to your computer, laptop, tablet or mobile device.
- If you have purchased this title as an e-book, access to your **Wiley E-Text** is available with proof of purchase within 90 days. Visit **http://support.wiley.com** and click on the 'Contact Support' tab.
- Open the Bookshelf application on your computer and register for an account.
- Follow the registration process and enter your redemption code to download your digital book.

The VitalSource Bookshelf can now be used to view your Wiley E-Text on iOS, Android and Kindle Fire!

- **For iOS:** Visit the app store to download the VitalSource Bookshelf: **http://bit.ly/17ib3XS**
- **For Android and Kindle Fire:** Visit the Google Play Market to download the VitalSource Bookshelf: **http://bit.ly/BSAAGP**

You can now sign in with the email address and password you used when you created your VitalSource Bookshelf Account

Full E-Text support for mobile devices is available at: **http://support. vitalsource.com**

PART 1

CHAPTER 1

Structured approach to acute psychiatric emergencies

Learning outcomes

After reading this chapter, you will be able to:

- Describe the approach to preparing for an assessment of a patient with possible mental health problems
- Explain the importance of close working between emergency medicine and psychiatry staff
- Outline the importance of good communication
- Identify a structured approach to managing psychiatric emergencies

---

1.1 Introduction

Psychiatric and behavioural presentations to Emergency Departments (EDs) are common. If substance misuse is included in the figures then some 35–40% of presentations (6–8 million each year in England) are defined as such. This means that on each shift staff are highly likely to have to manage patients with acute psychiatric and/or behavioural emergencies, and as will be explored below, they often do so with limited specialist training.

Adults with mental health illness are three times more likely to attend the ED and five times more likely to have a general admission to hospital (NICE and NHS England (2016)).

Systematic assessment and management of a person with acute mental health problems can present major challenges wherever they arise. Key considerations include:

Acute Psychiatric Emergencies: A Practical Approach, Second Edition.
Edited by Mark Buchanan and Damien Longson.
© 2025 John Wiley & Sons Ltd. Published 2025 by John Wiley & Sons Ltd.

- ED and acute hospital staff receive little training in managing psychiatric emergencies
- Responses of mental health staff can be delayed, inconsistent and unsystematic
- The acute hospital environment is rarely conducive to the provision of good psychiatric care

These considerations make clear the importance of the Acute Psychiatric Emergencies (APEx) course that seeks to provide a safe, practical system for practitioners. The approaches discussed in APEx are as relevant when seeing a patient in the ED as in any acute setting, including prehospital, the patient's home and prison. As such the APEx course is not just aimed at psychiatric and emergency medicine clinicians and allied professionals, but also at many other staff groups involved in the management of the patient who is presenting with a possible mental health emergency.

1.2 Preparation

Before starting any assessment for a patient with possible mental health problems:

- Gather any available information to allow you to make an assessment of the risk (to self and to the patient) and rapidly identify the need for emergency medical or psychiatric management using the Unified approach (ABCD/AEIO), which will be covered later in this chapter
- Ensure that appropriate help is available (a person who is showing signs of acute behavioural disturbance requires a team approach)
- Ensure there are suitable facilities to assess the patient

There must be a safe area where people who are acutely disturbed can be assessed and managed appropriately.

1.3 Close working between emergency and psychiatry staff

The safe and successful management of people with acute mental health problems requires close working between emergency/acute hospital teams and liaison mental health teams. Each team needs to carry out their own tasks, be aware of each other's skills and work collaboratively to ensure the best possible outcome.

1.4 Communication

Good communication and basic rapport building with a person with acute mental illness are essential. Communication is no less important with families of patients and with clinical colleagues – especially between those of different disciplines. Detailed records of current clinical findings, the patient's history, prior mental health records, physical test results and management plans must be completed, and communicated to staff who will be taking over the care of the patient when they leave the ED.

1.5   Consent

In an emergency, if it is deemed in the patient's best interests, hospital staff have a duty of care to treat the patient, provided treatment is limited to that which is reasonably required in that emergency situation.

As consent legislation is a complex area with different practices in different countries and jurisdictions, we will highlight the medicolegal aspects of patient care in relevant chapters by detailing the principles of what they achieve. Chapter 12 summarises legal aspects in more detail and maps the principles of the relevant laws. The details will differ depending on the jurisdictions where the APEx course is available.

1.6   A structured approach

A structured approach will enable all clinicians (whether mental health trained or not) to manage psychiatric emergencies optimally, so that patients receive high-quality care. It will also ensure that important steps in the care process are not forgotten. As it is common for mental and physical health problems to occur at the same time, both require consideration.

A structured approach focuses initially on a primary assessment designed to identify and manage any immediate threats to safety, either for the patient or for others. This involves a rapid assessment of physical risk – **Airway, Breathing, Circulation, Disability (ABCD)** – and a psychiatric risk assessment of **Agitation/ Arousal, Environment, Intent, Objects (AEIO)**. These then inform the **U**nified assessment.

After a primary assessment has been completed and relevant steps have been taken to ensure safety, a secondary assessment needs to be undertaken. This includes establishing the key features of the presentation. In particular, it is important to establish whether the presentation is predominantly a physical health or a mental health problem (or a combination of both). This process involves being able to interact with the patient in a manner that conveys understanding and empathy, builds rapport, reduces anxiety and enables information gathering in an effective and efficient manner. Secondary mental health assessment includes a focused conversational psychosocial history and examination of the mental state, while secondary physical health assessment involves a focused physical history and full top-to-toe examination. Following on from this, an appropriate emergency treatment and management plan can be implemented.

The final phase of the structured approach is to stabilise the patient so that transfer to an appropriate care environment can occur.

Throughout this text the same structure will be used so the clinician will become familiar with the approach and be able to apply it to any clinical emergency situation.

Figure 1.1 shows the structured approach in diagrammatic form.

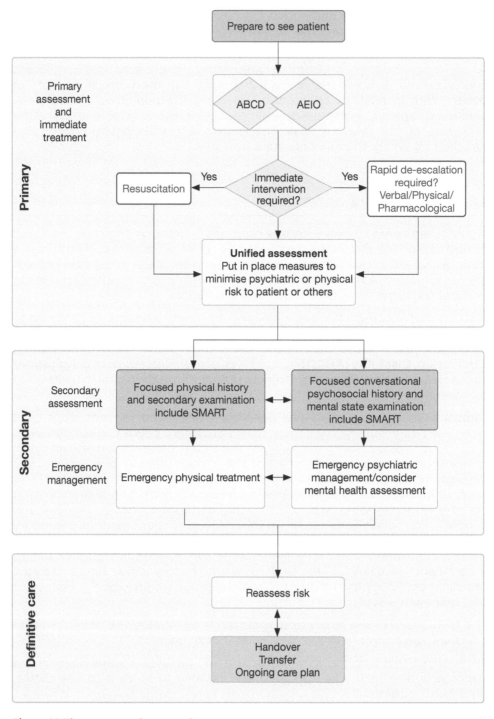

Figure 1.1 The structured approach
See Figure 3.2 for more detail on the SMART Form

1.7   Summary

This book will introduce the structured approach in more detail and then explore its use in the common psychosocial presentations to the ED.

CHAPTER 2

Primary unified assessment and immediate psychiatric management

---

Learning outcomes

After reading this chapter, you will be able to:

- Explain how to assess someone who is acutely disturbed
- Describe how to take structured steps to ensure safety and minimise any potential harm to others

---

2.1 Introduction

The effective management of an acutely disturbed patient who has a presumed mental health crisis is a key emergency skill. By using the basic techniques and strategies described, a safe framework can be established, from which a more detailed assessment or intervention can then be carried out. It is essential that all staff who work in an acute hospital setting have these basic skills.

In the structured approach, the person who is acutely disturbed should have a primary assessment that includes ABCD and AEIO risk assessments (see Figure 2.1). It may not be possible to carry out a full physical assessment because

---

Acute Psychiatric Emergencies: A Practical Approach, Second Edition.
Edited by Mark Buchanan and Damien Longson.
© 2025 John Wiley & Sons Ltd. Published 2025 by John Wiley & Sons Ltd.

of the level of disturbance, but consideration should be given to physical status and potential organic causes of the presentation.

In this chapter, we focus on the mental health assessment, but physical factors should always be considered and accompanied by a parallel physical assessment when appropriate.

2.2 Preparation

Never approach a patient who is acutely disturbed by yourself. Wait until a sufficient number of appropriately trained staff, police officers or security guards are present. The number required will depend upon the physical threat from the patient, the nature and degree of their disturbance, and the environment and resources of the facility in which you are working.

In most circumstances, there is time to gather information quickly before seeing the patient (e.g. if the patient is brought to the Emergency Department (ED) by the family, the police or the paramedic emergency service). The aim at this point is to access relevant information that will inform the rapid assessment.

Information may include verbal accounts from the family, paramedics, police, relevant others and the hospital record systems. Ask and obtain answers to the following questions:

- Can you tell me about the behaviour of X whilst in your care?
- On a 10 point scale (0 being not disturbed at all, to 10 being extremely agitated/violent/aroused) how would you rate this person's behaviour?
- Can you tell me about/give me an example of the most extreme or disturbed level of behaviour you have witnessed?
- Do they speak the local language and, if not, what language do they speak?

Many mental and physical health, social care and police record systems have specific, designated subsections for flagging information about 'risk of harm to self and others'. Attempts should be made to gain as much information about the patient as possible. Ensure all relevant information is shared between all staff involved with the patient.

Key factors to note are:

- A prior history of self-harm
- A prior history of harm to others
- Alcohol and illicit drug use
- Prior history of severe mental illness
- Prior history of violence, forensic history (mental health treatment in a secure setting because of criminal behaviour) or a criminal record

Table 2.1 AEIO assessment: minimum number of staff required for safe containment (this is suggested safety levels)

Arousal/agitation	Environment	Intent	Objects	Containment
Low	Low	Low	Low	Nil
Moderate	Low	Low	Low	One staff
Moderate	Moderate	Low	Low	Two staff
Moderate	Moderate	Low	Moderate	Three staff
Moderate	Moderate	Moderate	Low	Three staff
Moderate	Low	Moderate	Moderate	Three staff
High	Low	Low	Low	Three staff
High	Low	High	Low	Four staff
High	High	High	Low	Six staff
High	High	High	High	Six staff

Before entering a room with an agitated patient, make sure you have back-up in terms of available staff who can help if necessary. Have at least two other members of staff with you. There may already be staff or police officers in the room. Stay close to the door and keep it open. Do not allow yourself to be trapped behind the door. Consider the staffing recommendations in Table 2.1.

Make sure there is a way to sound an alarm, if needed, with a suitable response. Many 'safe rooms' in EDs do not have alarms because of inappropriate, frequent use. Make sure you have a personal attack alarm or that there is someone outside the room who can call for back-up.

It is usual for most patients to undergo triage from a member of the ED nursing staff soon after they present. However, if patients are either very physically unwell (for instance if they have stabbed themselves) or are significantly behaviorally disturbed, it may not be possible to do this. Do not assume that aggression or agitation is due to mental health issues; most aggression within acute settings is not related to a mental health crisis. Seek relevant physical health signs or symptoms that need to be addressed.

The structured approach is universally applicable to the management of all psychiatric emergencies in all settings and across the age spectrum.

2.3 Primary assessment: the Unified assessment

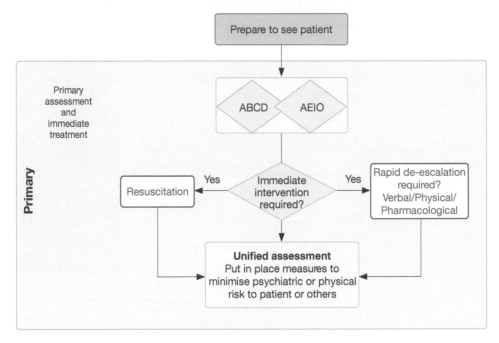

Prepare to see patient

Primary assessment and immediate treatment

Primary

ABCD   AEIO

Resuscitation   ← Yes ← Immediate intervention required? → Yes → Rapid de-escalation required? Verbal/Physical/ Pharmacological

Unified assessment
Put in place measures to minimise psychiatric or physical risk to patient or others

Figure 2.1 Structured approach: primary assessment

The first priority is to ensure that the patient is kept safe (both physically and psychologically) whilst they are awaiting detailed psychiatric assessment or are undergoing physical investigations. They must be prevented from either intentional or unintentional harming of themselves or others. A fast and focused assessment (Figure 2.1) is required to:

- Establish the level of physical and psychiatric risk using AEIO (see Section 2.5)
- Put in place appropriate measures to minimise that risk

Observe the patient. Note their conscious level, degree of agitation and current behaviour. When it is safe to do so introduce yourself:

- 'I'm X, I'm a doctor/nurse, I'm here to try and help you'
- Ask the patient their name and what they like to be called
- Ask them if they know where they are
- If they do not know, explain they are in a hospital, they are safe, and you are here to try and help them

As you are doing this, make a quick assessment of the patient's overt physical health. Look for skin colour (pallor or flushed), whether or not they are sweating, pupil size (pinpoint or dilated), any obvious injuries and any signs of self-harm (ligature mark around neck, scars to arms) or disabilities.

Ask the patient if they are hurt or in pain. If they respond positively, you will need to get details of their concerns to establish the nature of the injury or their physical health problems. Ask them if it would be okay for someone to check their pulse, temperature and blood pressure.

As you are doing this, make an assessment of their cognitive function, including basic orientation and attention.

- Can they give you their name and address and date of birth?
- Do they know where they are?
- Do they know the time of day, month and year?
- Do they understand questions?
- Do they respond appropriately?

Tell them that you need to ask them some brief questions to check that they are safe. Tell them that these are routine questions.

2.4   Primary physical risk assessment

The primary physical risk assessment should focus on four key areas:

ABCD

A **Airway**
patency and security

B **Breathing**
adequacy and effectiveness

C **Circulation**
adequacy

D **Disability**
assessment of conscious level and pupils

ABCD problems should be addressed as soon as they are identified. It is not in the scope of this book to describe the life support techniques that might be necessary – patients should be moved to the resuscitation area as soon as possible and physical resuscitation should be continued there whilst the AEIO assessment described below is carried out.

2.5 Primary psychiatric risk assessment

The primary psychiatric risk assessment should focus on four key areas:

AEIO

A **Agitation/Arousal** (current and highest reported level)

E **Environment** in which the patient is being cared for

I **Intent**/risk

O **Objects** that the patient has in their possession, which may be used for self-harm or harm to others

This enables staff to carry out a quick assessment of risk of harm (to self or others) and of flight risk. This enables planning of a risk reduction and containment strategy, which may or may not involve rapid tranquillisation.

A **Agitation/Arousal**

This assessment depends on a quick observation of the patient. Their level of arousal or agitation is determined according to the following guide. Ensure that you have considered the most agitated the patient is known to have been (either during this episode or in previous episodes) as well as their current state.

Level of arousal or agitation

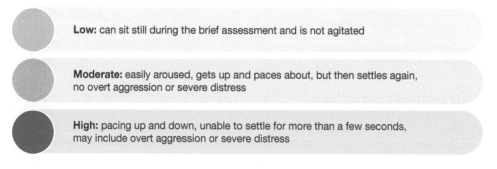

Low: can sit still during the brief assessment and is not agitated

Moderate: easily aroused, gets up and paces about, but then settles again, no overt aggression or severe distress

High: pacing up and down, unable to settle for more than a few seconds, may include overt aggression or severe distress

E **Environment**

All EDs should have facilities where an acutely disturbed person can be assessed and, if necessary, can be given emergency treatment.

Standards, for example those from the UK Royal College of Psychiatrists, suggest that EDs should only be used as a place of safety where medical problems need urgent assessment and management. However, many patients who are behaving in a disturbed manner may have underlying physical health problems, so will be brought to an ED.

Comparable facilities to those described here should therefore be available in every ED so patients with behavioural disturbance can be cared for safely. Box 2.1 describes the Royal College of Psychiatrists standards for place of safety rooms as outlined in Standards on the Use of Section 136 of the Mental Health Act 1983 (England and Wales) (CR159, 2011, Royal College of Psychiatrists).

Box 2.1 Standards for place of safety rooms

- The psychiatric assessment facility must be a lockable facility in order to be able to safely care for those who are disturbed*
- Levels of staff required to support this facility, when in use, are up to three staff trained in physical intervention, who should be available at short notice without compromising staffing levels and hence safety elsewhere. This is in addition to the staff carrying out the assessment
- The room should accommodate six people to allow both treatment and restraint, have an observation hatch and be lit well, have two outward opening doors at opposite ends of the room and have fixed, soft, comfortable chairs that cannot be used as a weapon. There should be no ligature points. In addition, a clock should be visible to both patients and staff, there should be a phone line with outside dialling, a panic alarm and CCTV. It should not be isolated and should be accessed easily for containment and restraint and resuscitation teams if required

* Note an acute trust is not a psychiatric assessment facility

In the absence of such a facility, or if it is already being used by another patient, make an assessment of the environment in which the patient is being contained. Note the following, using ADELLE as an acronym:

ADELLE

A	Alarm	Is there a panic alarm in the room?
D	Doors	Which way does the door (or doors) open?
E	Exits	How many exits are there, and how easy would it be for the patient to reach the exits from the room?
L	Ligature points	Identify any ligature points (including those in any bathroom or toilet facilities the patient may need to use)
L	Location	How isolated is the room from the rest of the ED or ward? Is there any CCTV? What floor are you on?
E	Equipment	Is there any equipment in the room (e.g. oxygen points, monitors) or on staff/team or items of furniture that could be used as a weapon or have sharp edges?

Never allow a patient who is disturbed, or whom you have concerns about, to be left alone in a room that has ligature points or equipment or furniture that could be used to self-harm.

Environmental risk assessment

Make an assessment of the environmental risk.

Environmental risk

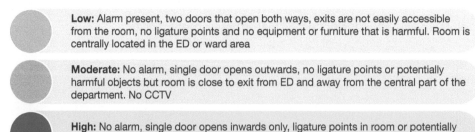

Low: Alarm present, two doors that open both ways, exits are not easily accessible from the room, no ligature points and no equipment or furniture that is harmful. Room is centrally located in the ED or ward area

Moderate: No alarm, single door opens outwards, no ligature points or potentially harmful objects but room is close to exit from ED and away from the central part of the department. No CCTV

High: No alarm, single door opens inwards only, ligature points in room or potentially harmful objects, etc.

Ⓘ Intent/risk

Intent involves assessment of the current and ongoing risks to the patient and to the staff. There are four aspects you need to assess quickly:

- Intent to harm themselves
- Intent to harm others
- Intent to leave the department
- Irrational thought (psychotic experiences)

Intent to harm themselves: current thoughts of harming self

Assess the nature, severity and frequency of these thoughts. Ask the patient directly how likely they are to act on these thoughts in the next couple of hours. Assess how able the patient is to resist these thoughts.

Intent to harm others: current thoughts of harm to others

Assess the nature, severity and frequency of these thoughts. Ask the patient how likely they are to act on these thoughts in the next few hours. Establish whether the thoughts of harm to others are based on a wish to inflict harm on others (possibly related to aggression) or are related to self-protection arising from fears of persecution. In the case of the former, a calm and non-confrontational approach may be helpful, whereas in the latter, active reassurance that the patient is safe and that staff are not going to harm them may reduce anxiety/agitation.

Intent to leave/abscond/desire to leave

Check whether the patient is willing to stay in the department until they can be more fully assessed. Note if the patient expresses thoughts about wanting to leave or if the patient has already tried to leave. Provide the patient with an estimate of how long they will need to stay in the department and explain to them what is likely to happen during this time (e.g. will they need more physical investigations, how long will the detailed psychiatric assessment take, etc.). Try to keep them informed and updated about what is happening.

Irrational thoughts: psychotic experiences

Certain psychotic experiences such as hearing voices commanding the patient to harm themselves, or others, or delusions of control can be associated with an increased risk of self-harm, harm to others or unpredictable behaviour.

Establish whether the patient appears to be responding to external stimuli or appears very agitated or frightened. If the level of agitation is too high than this may only be assessed by observing. When it is safe, try to access the patient's inner mental experiences by asking if anything is frightening or upsetting them or making them feel uneasy. Ask specifically about command hallucinations or delusions of control.

- *'Are you hearing anyone or anything telling you to harm yourself or others?'*
- *'Do you feel controlled in any way by anything, or made to do anything you don't want to do?'*

Intent assessment

Make an assessment of intent.

Intent assessment

Low: No suicidal ideas, or thoughts of harm to others, no command hallucinations or thoughts of wanting to leave

Moderate: Some thoughts of self-harm or thoughts of harming others, or thoughts of wanting to leave, but the patient can resist these thoughts

High: Thoughts of self-harm or harm to others that the patient finds difficult to resist. Appears to be responding to or experiencing hallucinations which the patient has described to have been commanding them to harm themself or others. Actively wants or is trying to leave

⊙ Objects on the patient

Establish whether the patient has any items on them or pieces of clothing that could either be used to harm themself or others. The obvious items are firearms, sharp objects such as scissors or razor blades, or other items such as medication, illicit drugs, plastic bags or batteries. Potentially harmful items of clothing include belts or scarves.

Take note of what the patient is wearing and, if they are willing, ask if they would consider removing any items of clothing that could be used to harm themselves (e.g. a belt or tie). Tell the patient you are doing your utmost to look after them and ensure they are safe. Ask the patient if they have anything else on them that they could use to harm themself, such as tablets or razor blades. Reassure the patient that their possessions will be kept safely for them.

The manner in which you broach these topics is more important than the actual words you use, and you will need to tailor your body language, tone of voice, phrasing and timing to each individual person according to their cue–response. Chapter 13 will focus in more depth on specific communication skills. Do **not** continue to ask questions if this process is increasing the patient's degree of agitation.

Risk from objects assessment

Make an assessment of risk from objects in the patient's possession.

Risk from objects

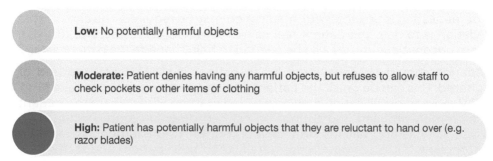

Low: No potentially harmful objects

Moderate: Patient denies having any harmful objects, but refuses to allow staff to check pockets or other items of clothing

High: Patient has potentially harmful objects that they are reluctant to hand over (e.g. razor blades)

2.6   Unified assessment and immediate treatment

You need to make a judgement as to the measures that need to be put in place to keep the patient safe in the department, based upon:

- Information you have gained about the patient
- Physical degree of agitation
- Current environment in which they are being contained
- Likelihood they still have items on them that they could use to harm themselves or others
- Their current suicidal intent (or other high-risk thoughts or behaviours)

By synthesising the ABCD/AEIO elements into an overall Unified risk assessment, you will be able to specify the degree of observation that is required (ranging from no additional measures to one-to-one, or several-to-one, constant observation) and the number of staff trained in physical intervention that need to be present either in the room or outside the room.

Table 2.1 provides a guide as to the minimum number of staff, trained in physical restraint, required according to the Unified assessment. There are no agreed published guidelines for staffing levels in such situations, and Table 2.1 has been reached by consensus agreement between the authors of the APEx course. The red boxes indicate levels of risk where you should be considering whether rapid tranquillisation will be necessary to keep the patient safe. Increase the number of members of staff required according to the size and level of agitation of the patient, and other relevant factors. Not all combinations of the AEIO are shown, but the examples included in Table 2.1 provide a quick reference guide.

Clinical judgement should always override the guidance in Table 2.1, which is a very basic starting point from which to plan care.

2.7 De-escalation, sedation and rapid tranquillisation

This is discussed in detail in Chapter 10.

De-escalation should always be the first step, before sedation and rapid tranquillisation.

If de-escalation is unsuccessful, medication may be required. The aim of rapid sedation is to help the patient feel calmer and less distressed, not to make them unconscious. It may also be needed to help manage the patient safely.

Sedation should be considered if the patient is significantly aroused or agitated. This can be oral if the patient is willing but response can take time. IM/IV rapid tranquillisation may be needed in some cases where the patient is extremely aroused and cannot be calmed down. It is used when both psychological approaches and environmental management have been insufficient. If it is delivered parenterally then both patient and staff safety should be paramount. It is important to follow your hospital protocol. All patients who have been sedated require regular monitoring (at least hourly or more frequently if consciousness is impaired).

2.8 Staff safety

If you find yourself alone with an acutely disturbed patient, do not approach them. Keep your distance (at least two arms' length away). Locate the nearest exit and make your way towards it. Tell the patient your name, tell them you are a member of staff and you are going to get some more help for them. Speak in a calm voice and keep looking at the patient, but do not make intense eye contact. Do not turn your back. As soon as you can, leave via the exit and shout for help.

If you are concerned you are going to be attacked:

- Use your personal alarm if you have one
- Use the hospital alarm system, if one is installed and you can reach it
- Shout for help
- Try to run or get away

If you are caught or grabbed by the patient, you may have to use basic techniques to release yourself. There are many courses available that offer training in these skills.

2.9 Person-centred care

All patients and healthcare professionals have rights and responsibilities. The focus in this chapter has been on the need to conduct a primary physical and psychiatric assessment to keep someone safe in the emergency situation, whilst further physical or mental health assessments are undertaken.

This does not remove the need to adopt a patient-centred, trauma-informed, values-based approach to care. The patient's rights are respected and efforts are made to develop a trusting therapeutic relationship. It has been shown that dedicated mental health support workers, whose role is to provide reassurance, listen and engage with patients who are contained in a room for their own safety, can have a positive impact upon the patient's experience. Such workers can explain any legal processes, help to de-escalate tension or aggression, provide basic comforts such as food or drink, and help the patient to contact family members or friends.

2.10   Legal framework

The legal framework under which staff provide assessment and care for patients with acute behavioural disturbance in the emergency situation will vary depending on the nature of the person's disturbance and their pathway through the crisis. A discussion of the legal framework, which covers acute psychiatric emergencies, is given in Chapter 12.

2.11   Secondary assessment

Once steps have been put in place to minimise the risk of harm to the patient or others, the ED and psychiatric team should work collaboratively to undertake a parallel physical and full mental health assessment. In the UK this is usually the psychiatric liaison team. The aim is to determine the most likely cause of the patient's disturbance and the most appropriate facility to which the person should be admitted. In most cases the degree of disturbance will warrant admission to either a medical ward or mental health facility.

2.12   Summary

It is important to use a structured ABCD/AEIO Unified approach to the assessment of someone who is acutely disturbed to ensure their safety and minimise any potential harm to others.

CHAPTER 3

Secondary physical and psychosocial assessment

Learning outcomes

After reading this chapter, you will be able to:

- Describe how to apply the structured approach to a combined secondary physical and psychosocial assessment
- Explain the structure of a focused conversational psychosocial history

---

3.1 Introduction

In this chapter, we will explore the secondary assessment of potential physical and psychosocial factors, which may be contributing to the acute mental health emergency. This element of the structured approach is shown in Figure 3.1.

> **Key point: background information**
>
> Prior to the secondary assessment, obtain maximum background information where possible. This can be done personally or with the support of a colleague. Sources include:
>
> - Directly from paramedics or those involved in sending the patient to hospital
> - The patient's records (health care, social care, police) for background information prior to the secondary assessment
> - Family members, friends, etc.

Acute Psychiatric Emergencies: A Practical Approach, Second Edition.
Edited by Mark Buchanan and Damien Longson.
© 2025 John Wiley & Sons Ltd. Published 2025 by John Wiley & Sons Ltd.

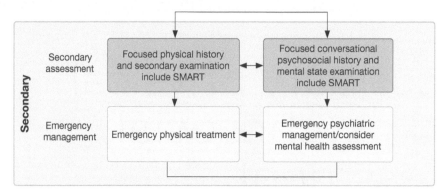

Figure 3.1 Structured approach: secondary assessment

3.2   SMART triage

It is essential as part of the triage to identify any physical issues early. This may expedite any investigations required and reduce the risk of diagnostic overshadowing. Diagnostic overshadowing is when symptoms are attributed to a psychiatric problem rather than to a coexisting or independent physical problem.

The SMART Form (Figure 3.2) is a useful aid to reduce the risk of diagnostic overshadowing. It is a medical clearance tool used in the USA to help prevent unnecessary delays in the care of a patient attending the ED with a presumed mental health related presentation. The tool highlights areas in the history or observations that may increase the likelihood of a physical problem, and might suggest the need for investigations and more in depth physical assessment.

The SMART Form (Figure 3.2) is further discussed in Chapter 7.

SMART

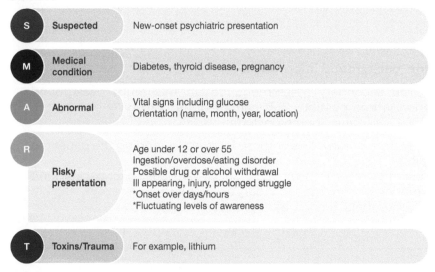

S	Suspected	New-onset psychiatric presentation
M	Medical condition	Diabetes, thyroid disease, pregnancy
A	Abnormal	Vital signs including glucose Orientation (name, month, year, location)
R	Risky presentation	Age under 12 or over 55 Ingestion/overdose/eating disorder Possible drug or alcohol withdrawal Ill appearing, injury, prolonged struggle *Onset over days/hours *Fluctuating levels of awareness
T	Toxins/Trauma	For example, lithium

* Not in the original form but seen as a risky presentation

Figure 3.2 SMART clearance tool
Source: Adapted from Sierra Sacramento Valley Medical Society: smartmedical clearance.org

3.3   History: general principles

Allow the patient to talk freely initially, telling you what has happened and what led to them coming into hospital. A conversational style should be adopted. Commonly, this initial opening interaction will reveal many of the symptoms contributing to the presentation.

The history should include the presenting complaint, a focused physical and psychiatric history, relevant physical and mental health and forensic history (Figure 3.3). Medication history should be noted. This should include alcohol and substances of misuse. Social history is important, including housing, family and friend support networks. When appropriate, emotional trauma and/or adverse childhood experiences (ACEs) may be explored.

PHRASED

	Focused physical history	Focused conversational psychosocial history
P	Presenting complaint	Problem
H	History of presenting complaint	History of presenting psychiatric problem, e.g. SLIPA
R	Relevant medical history	Relevant psychiatric and forensic history
A	Allergies	Allergies
S	Systems review	Substance (mis)use and self-harm
E	Essential family and social history	Emotional trauma
D	Drugs	Drugs

Figure 3.3 PHRASED approach
SLIPA, **S**uicidal thoughts at the time of self-harm, **L**ethality of the episode, **I**ntent now, **P**rotective factors, **A**dverse factors

3.4 Focused physical history and examination

The principal aims of the focused physical history and examination are to:

- Identify any physical elements potentially contributing to the acute psychiatric presentation and determine the need for emergency treatment
- Identify any physical sequelae of the mental health emergency that will require treatment, e.g. self-harm wounds, overdose, ingested objects
- Determine the pre-existing physical health status of the patient

> **Before making a diagnosis of a primary psychiatric disorder, consider whether alternative physical causes are contributing to the presentation. The psychiatric team may still have a key role in the initial assessment.**

Many physical illnesses may present with psychiatric symptoms, particularly if it is a first presentation. If the patient has an established diagnosis of a major mental illness, the likelihood of organic illness is reduced but must still be considered.

A pragmatic approach should be adopted, making best use of available history and permitted examination. The vast majority of patients presenting in psychiatric crisis may be examined safely and adequately, once they feel safe. Ideally, a full secondary assessment (incorporating a comprehensive history and systems enquiry, together with a head-to-toe physical examination) would determine the physical health status, but usually is neither necessary nor practical.

Therefore, attempt to de-escalate an acutely agitated patient during history taking. Physical examination requires close proximity and the clinician should make a risk assessment before commencing. One technique is to persuade the patient to permit basic observations, then ease into direct physical examination. In extreme circumstances, it may be necessary to use medication (sedation, tranquillisation) prior to examination.

The physical examination for the secondary assessment of patients in psychiatric crisis is outlined in the relevant chapters of this book. Physical investigations will be determined by history and examination.

> **There is no standard investigation panel for mental health emergency presentations, and no specific tests mandated to 'physically clear' the patient.**

3.5 Focused conversational psychosocial history

The principal aims of the psychosocial history, at this stage, are to:

- Engage in dialogue with the patient to aid de-escalation of the emergency
- Identify key factors contributing to presentation
- Further explore and review factors that may influence assessment of capacity when and if decisions will be required
- Consider non-organic ('functional') symptoms indicating possible need for referral to an acute psychiatric service

Questions to consider include:

- *'Have you harmed yourself in any way?'*
- *'Have you swallowed any tablets or anything else that might be harmful in the last 24–48 hours?'*
- *'Have you had any alcohol?'*
- *'Have you taken any drugs (also asking about novel psychoactive substances, cocaine, cannabis, ketamine, medicines that are prescribed for other people)'*
- *'Have you suffered a recent head injury?''*

If self-harm or overdose has happened, then a SLIPA assessment (see Chapter 6) is helpful as it helps identify current risks and safety systems that may be present.

SLIPA

S	Suicidal thoughts at the time of self-harm
L	Lethality of the episode
I	Intent now
P	Protective factors
A	Adverse factors

3.6   Secondary psychosocial (mental state) examination

See Chapter 4.

3.7   Summary

This chapter has outlined both the physical secondary assessments. The elements of the structured approach will be explored in more detail in the context of specific patient presentations in the following chapters.

Mental state examination

Learning outcomes

After reading this chapter, you will be able to:

- Define the parts of the mental state examination
- Describe the psychopathology of psychiatric emergency care

4.1 Introduction

Assessment of a patient's mental state is something that happens throughout or even before the consultation. It is not necessarily a separate process. The complete assessment may not be done in a specified order or achieved with any particular questions. It will be built up from conversation with the patient, although some specific questions may be required, for example about the presence of delusions or hallucinations.

4.2 Mental state examination

The mental state examination consists of both verbal and non-verbal elements. Even if the patient is unable, or unwilling, to give a coherent history or engage in the assessment, many of the aspects of the mental state examination can be obtained from observation of the patient.

The mental state examination may be structured using the mnemonic ASEPTIC (Figure 4.1 and Box 4.1).

Acute Psychiatric Emergencies: A Practical Approach, Second Edition.
Edited by Mark Buchanan and Damien Longson.

ASEPTIC

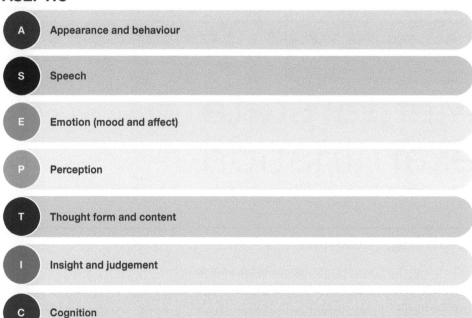

A Appearance and behaviour

S Speech

E Emotion (mood and affect)

P Perception

T Thought form and content

I Insight and judgement

C Cognition

Figure 4.1 ASEPTIC assessment

Box 4.1 ASEPTIC assessment

1. (A)PPEARANCE AND BEHAVIOUR

Apparent age	Stated age? Younger/older?
Dress	Casually, formally, poorly?
Grooming	Good or poor?
Hygiene	Good or poor?
Gait	Brisk, slow, intoxicated, ataxic, rigid, shuffling, staggering, uncoordinated?
Psychomotor activity	Normal, reduced, excessive?
Abnormal movements	Grimaces, tics, tardive dyskinesia, foot tapping, ritualistic behaviour?
Eye contact	Good or poor?
Attitude	Cooperative, belligerent, oppositional, submissive, etc.?

2. (S)PEECH

Rate	Rapid, pressured, slowed?
Rhythm	Hesitant, rambling, halting, stuttering, jerky, long pauses?
Tone of voice	Appropriate or inappropriate tone of voice?
Volume	Loud, soft, whispered, yelling, inaudible?
Accent	Any accent?
Clarity	Pronunciation, articulation?
Quantity	Responds only to questions, offers information, repetitive, verbose?

3. (E)MOTION (mood and affect)

Mood: patient's subjective emotional state	When the clinician asks, '*How is your mood?*' and the patient responds, '*Good*', '*Depressed*', '*Down*', etc.
Affect: objective emotional state	What you actually observe about how they appear to be feeling, e.g. if their affect appears down, euphoric, etc.
Congruence to mood/ appropriateness	Congruent mood means that the mood is appropriate to the situation, e.g. patient's father has passed away and the patient is sad Incongruent mood means that the mood is inappropriate to the situation, e.g. patient's father has passed away and the patient is laughing
Quality	Euthymic, elevated, depressed?
Range	Broad/restricted?
Stability	Fixed/labile?

4. (P)ERCEPTION

Hallucinations	Auditory: '*Have you heard any things that others can't hear?*' Visual: '*Have you seen any things that others can't hear?*' Olfactory: '*Any unusual smells that you notice, e.g. burning smells?*'
Illusions	Distortions of real images or sensations
Depersonalisation	Patient feels that they are not real Clinician: '*Do you ever feel that you are not real?*'
Derealisation	Patient feels that the world is not real Clinician: '*Do you ever feel that things around you aren't real?*'

5. (T)HOUGHT FORM AND CONTENT

Thought process	How well are the patient's thoughts connected? Are the patient's thoughts coherent, logical, relevant? Does the patient tend to go off topic? (e.g. circumstantial) Does the patient completely go from one thing to the next? (e.g. tangential (as in mania, psychoses); flight of ideas (as in mania, disconnecting rambling from one idea to the next); loosening of associations (as in psychosis with shifting from one subject to another) Word salad (as in schizophrenia, with seemingly random words and phrases) Echolalia (as in Tourette's where patient copies another's speech) Neologisms (as in psychosis with patient making up new words)

Thought content	
Delusions*	Delusions (to friends and family): *'Does your loved one have any strong or unusual beliefs?'* Delusions (to the patient) *'Everyone has beliefs. Some people are religious. Some people believe in UFOs. Some people believe that the government is spying on us. Do you have any strong beliefs?'* Paranoid delusions: *'Do you feel that people are watching you, following you or trying to hurt you?'* Delusions of grandeur: *'Do you have any special powers or skills?'*
Suicidal ideation	*'With all the stress that you've been under, has it ever got to the point that you feel life isn't worth living?'* If positive, then ask: *'What's the strongest those thoughts have been?'*; *'At this moment, do you have any thoughts of ending your life?'*
Homicidal ideation	*'Any thoughts of hurting other people?'*

6. (I)NSIGHT AND JUDGEMENT

Insight	Assuming the patient has difficulties and/or an illness, does the patient understand this? Good insight: patient understands they are ill and need treatment Partial insight may indicate that the patient acknowledges a problem, but is not willing to seek appropriate help or treatment Poor insight means that the patient does not see that they are ill nor does the patient need any help or treatment
Judgement	Is patient able to use facts and make reasonable decisions? May be good, fair, impaired

7. (C)OGNITION

Level of consciousness	Alert, confused, lethargic, stuporous
Orientation in three spheres	Name: *'What is your name?'* Place: *'Where are you right now?'* Time: *'What year, month, day is it?'*
Attention/ concentration	How well does the patient seem to be able to focus?

| Memory | How well can the patient remember? Short term: can the patient recall recent things that have happened? Long term: can the patient recall distant events? |
| Intelligence (globally and intellectual functions) | Based on your observations and patient's use of speech, does the patient's overall intelligence and cognition appear to be: (i) below average; (ii) average; or (iii) above average? |

*Note: Delusion is 'a false fixed belief that is not amenable to change in light of conflicting evidence, and outside of cultural and societal norms for that patient.'

Source: Reproduced with permission of eMentalHealth.ca: https://primary care.ementalhealth.ca/index.php?m=fpArticle&ID=26974

A Appearance and behaviour

Observe the patient, assessing appearance and behaviour:

- Clothing
- Abnormal movements
- Activity
- Rapport, including aggression

Clothing: what are they wearing?

- Old, worn or inappropriate clothing for the weather may indicate diagnoses such as psychotic illness, mania, severe depression, alcohol/substance misuse and dementia
- Bright or inappropriate clothing (e.g. bright clothes, sunglasses on a rainy day, tin foil on their head) may indicate mania, acute psychosis, etc.

Abnormal movements: is the patient moving strangely?

- Abnormal movements are often non-specific but may indicate organic or functional pathology
- Look for tics, movements of the mouth or tongue, and abnormal movements of the upper and lower limbs
- Chronic schizophrenia may result in movement disorders such as echopraxia, stereotypies, mannerisms, posturing or negativism
- Fidgeting with hair, clothes or nails may be seen in patients with anxiety disorders or substance misuse
- Scratching themselves, repeatedly banging their head against the wall and rocking may be reactions to severe distress but are also seen in learning disability
- Looking toward unseen objects, or responding to unseen stimuli, may indicate hallucinatory experiences

Activity: how active are they?

- Underactivity (psychomotor retardation): this may be seen in severe depression, severe physical illness including head injury, and intoxication with both drugs and alcohol. Stupor is an extreme example where the patient is mute with complete immobility
- Overactivity (psychomotor agitation): this may be due to mania, anxiety, acute drug intoxication, acute confusional state or head injury. Akathisia is agitation and restlessness due to neuroleptic medication

Rapport: how does the patient relate to you?

- Overfamiliarity may be due to frontal lobe damage, intoxication or mania. Difficulty in forming a rapport may be seen in severe depression. Psychotic patients may appear suspicious, frightened, guarded or reluctant to give you information
- Aggression: this may be a symptom of many different conditions and is not necessarily pathological

S Speech

Assess the rate and form of the speech. If abnormal, exclude underlying problems such as deafness, previous stroke or not using their mother tongue.

Reduced volume and rate of speech may be related to several disorders, including cerebrovascular accident, severe depression, schizophrenia and learning difficulties. Patients may talk rapidly, loudly or be difficult to interrupt in cases of intoxication, mania, anxiety and hypomania.

E Emotion (mood and affect)

Assess the patient's mood, e.g. depressed, elated or irritable. Ask how they feel (subjective mood) and note what you see (objective mood). Is it appropriate (congruent) or not (incongruent) for the situation? Mood may affect the patient's ability to weigh up information and therefore impact on their ability to make capacitous decisions.

P Perception (hallucinations and illusions)

Hallucinations are perceptions in the *absence* of a stimulus.

Hallucinations may occur in any sensory modality (taste, smell, touch, sight and hearing). They are not usually part of a normal human experience and should be considered as significant in almost all cases.

Auditory hallucinations (often 'voices') are generally non-diagnostic – they are almost ubiquitous in delirium, occur commonly in other organic disorders and are frequent in a wide range of psychotic disorders. Hallucinations in the other sensory modalities should significantly raise suspicion of organic disorders or intoxication with illicit drugs.

Illusions are the misinterpretation of a *real* stimulus.

Some illusions arise in mood states such as anxiety (e.g. misperceiving a shadow as a potential assailant).

Ⓣ Thoughts

Assessment of thought is complex and is dependent on obtaining a history. Two aspects should be assessed: **form** and **content**.

Disorders of thought: form

This should be suspected when the patient's responses to your questions are not making sense.

Examples of disorders of thought include:

- Circumstantiality (lots of unnecessary detail)
- Tangential thinking (answer moves focus away from the question)
- Loosening of associations (strange or absent associations between elements of speech)
- Neologism (made-up words)
- Flight of ideas
- Perseveration
- Echolalia (the patient immediately repeats your speech)
- Slow, simplified thoughts and thought block

Finding of any of these symptoms is significant.

Disorders of thought: content

In general, thoughts are either non-psychotic or psychotic and may be organic or non-organic.

Non-psychotic thoughts may be hypochondriacal, catastrophic, depressive, obsessional, phobic etc.

Psychotic thoughts are frequently frightening, unusual experiences that are almost always abnormal.

Examples of psychotic thoughts:

- Delusions: false and unshakeable beliefs that are held contrary to the patient's normal culture and experiences
- Delusions of control and passivity phenomena: some aspects of the patient's sensorium (thoughts, feelings, movements and sensations) are being controlled by an external agency
- Overvalued ideas: ideas that are unreasonable and strongly maintained with many elements of a delusional belief. However, the patient is able to recognise that the idea may not be true or culturally appropriate

Ⓘ Insight and capacity/judgement

Explore the patient's understanding of their symptoms, illness, investigations or treatment being offered. Insight may affect the patient's ability to weigh up information and therefore impact on their ability to make capacitous decisions.

> **Insight and capacity for any specific decisions must be carefully documented. Also document thoroughly any actions taken in the patient's best interests for those patients who are judged not to have capacity.**

Ⓒ Cognition

Psychiatric emergencies commonly have an organic contribution, with degrees of impairment of consciousness as a significant contributory factor to the behavioural disturbance. Secondary assessment in a mental health emergency should include assessment for orientation in time, place and person. Chapter 9 deals with assessment and management of a patient if delirium/acute confusional state is suspected.

4.3 Summary

ASEPTIC is a helpful mnemonic to aid the assessment of the mental state.

ASEPTIC can also be used to structure communication of the mental state during handover of care: situation, background, assessment and recommendation (SBAR).

The elements of the structured approach will be explored in more detail in the context of specific patient presentations in the following chapters.

CHAPTER 5

Commonly encountered psychiatric presentations

Learning outcomes

After reading this chapter, you will be able to:

- Discuss commonly encountered pyschiatric presentations of schizophrenia, drug-induced psychosis, catatonia, bipolar affective disorder, depression, intoxication and withdrawal, delerium and dementia, anxiety, dissociative disorders, and personality disorder

---

5.1   Introduction

In this chapter we will explore some common mental health diagnoses that may present as psychiatric emergencies.

5.2   Schizophrenia

This is a very heterogeneous disorder but the core symptoms must have been present for at least 1 month (any illness fulfilling the criteria but present for less than a month is classed as an acute schizophrenia-like psychotic disorder).

Acute Psychiatric Emergencies: A Practical Approach, Second Edition.
Edited by Mark Buchanan and Damien Longson.
© 2025 John Wiley & Sons Ltd. Published 2025 by John Wiley & Sons Ltd.

Schizophrenia is a functional psychosis that does not affect the level of consciousness and is characterised by five groups of symptoms:

- Delusions
- Hallucinations
- Disorganised speech
- Grossly disorganised behaviour
- Negative symptoms

There may also be subtle but generalised cognitive impairments that are stable over years. These typically produce impairments in performance without the relatively severe problems with orientation, amnesia or judgement common in dementia.

5.3 Drug-induced psychosis, psychotic episodes and delusional disorders

These disorders all include various features of schizophrenia with delusions and/or hallucinations but the symptoms demonstrated would fail to meet the full diagnostic criteria for schizophrenia.

5.4 Catatonia

Psychiatric emergencies can present with signs of catatonia, although these are often missed. Catatonia can be associated with a mental disorder such as schizophrenia, mood disorders and neurodevelopmental disorders. It can also be associated with intoxication with or withdrawal from psychoactive substances, or be secondary to an organic illness. For a diagnosis of secondary catatonia syndrome, the disorder must be a direct pathophysiological consequence of a medical condition or physical cause.

Diagnosis is dependent on three or more of the following symptoms: stupor, catalepsy, waxy flexibility, mutism, negativism, posturing, mannerism, sterotypy, agitation, grimacing, echolalia and echopraxia.

5.5 Bipolar affective disorder

Mania or hypomania commonly presents with overactivity, pressure of speech, flight of ideas and disinhibited behaviour. Patients may present as irritable or aggressive. If delusions and hallucinations are present they are termed as mood congruent, such as a belief that the person has special powers such as being able to fly or has God-like abilities. Patients with full-blown mania may be easy to spot purely by their appearance – for example, wearing brightly coloured shorts and T-shirt with sunglasses in the middle of winter.

Episodes of depression are discussed below.

Mixed states involve features of both elation and depression, or rapid shifts in affect that can lead to striking shifts in mental state and behaviour.

5.6   Depression

The mental states associated with depression often seem understandable. They are unlikely to seem strange unless the depression is severe and may be associated with severe retardation and poverty of thought. The patient may also ruminate on stereotyped depressive themes. Severe depression can lead to psychotic features with the presence of delusions and hallucinations, which are typically mood congruent. Sometimes severe anxiety (see below) can be a prominent feature

5.7   Intoxication and withdrawal

Intoxication and withdrawal from alcohol and drugs of misuse can present with many psychiatric symptoms including depression, anxiety and psychosis. These symptoms may be short lived or lead to ongoing psychiatric illness.

See Chapter 8.

5.8   Delirium and dementia

Delirium is seen as a sudden alteration to mental state. It is usually a consequence of an insult such as illness, medication or injury.

Dementia is a syndrome associated with a decline in brain function that affects thinking, language, memory, mood and behaviour.

See Chapter 9.

5.9   Anxiety

This is likely to be understandable unless severe agitation affects behaviour, or repetitive worries lead patients to behave oddly and to have difficulty participating in the assessment process. Patients will often somatise acutely during panic attacks – e.g. complain of choking, being hot, breathless, physically distressed or other isolated symptoms. When such somatisation is part of the history rather than the mental state (i.e. they present after they have recovered), then hypochondriacal ideation or somatisation may be less obvious.

5.10   Dissociative disorders, functional neurological disorders and PTSD

These occur when patients are unable to use some aspect of their normal automatic central nervous system (CNS) functions, such as movement, sensation, etc. This happens when patients experience a severe stress, although when they have happened once, less severe stresses can precipitate a recurrence. A key to diagnosing these syndromes is to identify the stressor and a timeline link to the physical symptoms.

A history of trauma is not necessary for diagnosis, and diagnosis of FND should be made based on clinical history and signs. During acute, stress-induced dissociation patients can often feel 'numb' and experience the world as somehow distant – think of the opening scene of the film *Saving Private Ryan* for a representation of this state. Patients can appear to be distant, 'mechanical' and have limited attention and difficulty integrating with function. This state may be relieved if patients instead experience a more isolated, specific CNS dysfunction, including paralysis, numbness or amnesia – they may seem oddly unconcerned, '*a belle indifference*'.

These states, particularly acute dissociative 'numbness', may have some relation to post-traumatic syndromes such as post-traumatic stress disorder (PTSD), where states marked by dissociation and numbness alternate with re-experiencing the trauma, including arousal, agitation, lability, dreams and hallucinations.

5.11   Personality disorder

Personality disorders predispose a person to most other forms of mental disorder, so they can lead to unusual behaviour through a range of mechanisms. However, those with features of histrionic personality disorder can present with dramatic accounts of, and reactions to, otherwise typical problems. Those with dissocial or emotionally unstable traits are more likely to malinger or present with factitious and other related disorders. Meeting the needs of patients with personality disorders can be difficult in the emergency situation.

PART 2

CHAPTER 6

The patient who has harmed themselves

Learning outcomes

After reading this chapter, you will be able to:

- Describe how the structured approach can be applied to patients who have self-harmed
- Perform a mental health assessment in patients who have self-harmed
- Identify how to integrate the mental health assessment with the physical healthcare of the patient with self-harm

---

6.1 Introduction

There are 200 000 presentations per year to Emergency Departments (EDs) in England following self-harm (*Hospital Episode Statistics* and *Emergency Care Data Set*, NHS England Digital). Not all people who self-harm have suicidal intent, but self-harming behaviour is linked with a 30-fold increase in the risk of future completed suicide, as compared with the general population. There is also a high prevalence of psychiatric morbidity in those who self-harm, with over 80% suffering from one or more types (e.g. depression, anxiety disorders). Between 15% and 30% of people will repeat self-harm within a 12-month period, and these people are at even higher risk of suicide.

Many people who attend an ED following self-harm report negative attitudes from hospital staff, which may cause an unnecessary increase in their distress. This may arise from a lack of understanding of the nature of emotional pain (which can be as severe as or even more distressing than physical pain), a lack of awareness of the high risk of eventual suicide of such patients, or a lack of training of emergency staff to appropriately manage patients who present with self-harm.

Acute Psychiatric Emergencies: A Practical Approach, Second Edition.
Edited by Mark Buchanan and Damien Longson.

Many people who self-harm have suffered adverse childhood experiences including abuse and neglect and many have led difficult and challenging lives. They are an extremely vulnerable group of people who find it difficult to cope with adversity.

Approximately 40% of people who die by suicide in England attend an ED in the year prior to death. The majority of these attendances are either for self-harm or a request for help with their mental health. Individuals who attend on multiple occasions for mental health reasons or for self-harm are at particularly high risk of suicide. Clinicians should therefore be alert to the risk associated with such presentations and be able to assess and treat patients according to their risk profile and mental health needs.

6.2   General principles

National Institute for Health and Care Excellence (NICE) guidelines have suggested some general principles for all healthcare professionals when helping people who have self-harmed (NICE Guideline NG225, 2022):

- Treat the person with respect, dignity and compassion, with an awareness of cultural sensitivity
- Take account of the person's emotional and mental state and level of distress
- When involving family members or carers in supporting a person who has self-harmed, give them opportunities to be involved in decision making, care planning and developing Safety Plans

Remember to involve the person who has self-harmed in clinical decision making and provide information about treatment options.

6.3   Preparation

People who self-harm require assessment of both their physical and mental health. Whenever possible this should be conducted in a flexible and fluid way, to increase efficiency and minimise any distress to the patient. It involves close, collaborative working between ED staff and mental health liaison teams, with each member of staff facilitating the work of others.

If the patient is acutely physically ill, medical care should follow a structured approach with a focus on primary physical assessment, with resuscitation, if necessary. A secondary mental health assessment is not practical, feasible or indeed a priority in these circumstances.

Most patients will undergo a form of triage when they attend the ED; either as part of this process, or immediately following it, a primary (AEIO) assessment must be carried out. This should include a plan for immediate management within the department, which specifies the degree of observation required to keep the patient safe. In the case of the acutely ill patient, this assessment should occur as soon as they are physically stable and conscious. Figure 6.1 shows the pathway that most patients will follow within the ED, depending upon their risk status and whether they are intimating that they wish to leave.

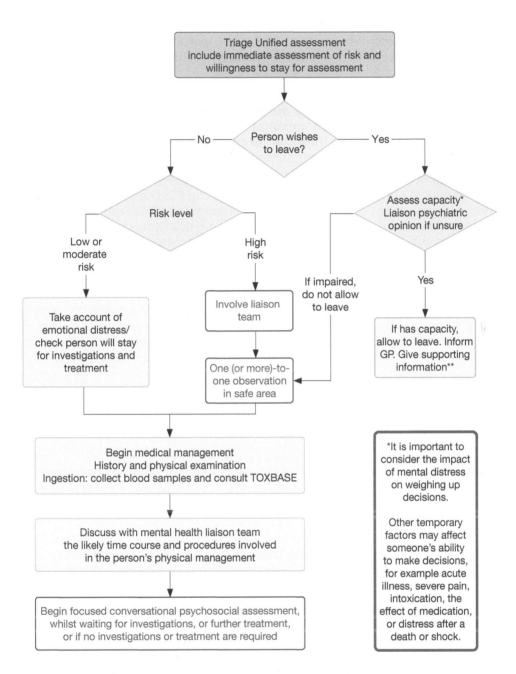

Figure 6.1 ED pathway for patients who have harmed themselves

The AEIO risk assessment can fluctuate. It is important to reassess following a change in environment or handover of care, or change in condition of the patient.

> **Patients can and do die by suicide in the acute hospital setting (either in the ED or on hospital wards), or leave the hospital precipitiously with the intention of taking their own lives.**

If the patient is transferred from the ED to an acute ward or intensive care unit before an assessment has taken place in the ED, the patient should be assessed as soon as possible in the new environment. It may only be possible to carry out a brief assessment of immediate risk at this stage, but a plan regarding the level of observation the patient requires must be written in the medical notes and conveyed to all relevant staff. It should not be assumed that because the patient is still physically unwell, they are free from risk of further self-harm.

Mental health staff should **not** wait until the patient is medically fit before carrying out an assessment. Where possible, patients should be seen jointly by the medical and psychiatric teams. Risk needs to be reviewed and managed as soon as the patient is conscious, followed by a more detailed assessment when the patient is capable of participating more fully. This has been supported by the *Side by Side* document agreed by the Royal College of Psychiatrists (RCPsych), Royal College of Emergency Medicine (RCEM), Royal College of Physicians (RCP) and Royal College of Nursing (RCN). This is backed up by the NICE self-harm guidance.

If immediate medical management is not required to save life, a more integrated physical and mental health assessment should be conducted. A common error in the management of self-harm is to delay mental health assessment until all medical treatment is completed.

6.4   Primary assessment: the Unified assessment

Before any physical investigations are carried out, establish the following:

- Immediate or short-term risk of further self-harm or suicide or harm to others (AEIO and SLIPA (see later in this chapter))
- Likelihood of the patient leaving the ED before physical and mental health assessment can be carried out

Put in place measures to mitigate risk if either is deemed to be high, as outlined in Chapter 2. Use this structured approach if the patient is highly aroused, agitated, aggressive or actively trying to leave the department. The following discussion assumes that the patient is relatively calm and is able to participate in the triage process, as is the case for the overwhelming majority of people who self-harm. The approach follows the basic principles of AEIO, but is specifically tailored for people who have self-harmed.

Triage: risk of further self-harm or suicide

As part of the triage process practitioners will need to prioritise the patient with self-harm for further clinical assessment. This will require an integrated approach to the assessment of physical and psychiatric risk.

A recognised tool should be used such as the Manchester Triage System (MTS) *Emergency Triage*, 3rd edn version 3.8 (2023). The MTS offers a range of charts specific to mental health presentations, including the self-harm algorithm (Figure 6.2).

In 2022, following an extensive international multiprofessional Delphi study, 19 new mental health discriminators were added, representing the biggest change in MTS since the original development of the first edition in 1996. The new discriminators have been added across all priorities, most significantly ensuring there are now Red (P1, immediate) discriminators to rapidly identify life-threatening mental health emergencies. The most important aspect of these additions is that MTS now has parity of esteem for both physical and mental health presentations.

Emergency nurses are well versed in assessing physical risk such as that of breathing difficulties in someone with an insecure airway. They may be less experienced in the assessment of risk of further self-harm during the brief triage assessment.

Questions about risk are best asked in context, when gathering information about what the person has actually done to harm themselves. However, triage is a rapid assessment and assignment of priority and deciding to ask clarifying questions should be balanced against the triage event becoming more of a lengthy consultation resulting in a delay for other patients requiring triage.

If clarifying questions are appropriate, it may be useful to ask the patient the following:

> *'And when you took the tablets (or cut your throat, etc.), what thoughts were in your mind at the time?'*

Staff should note how the patient responds and, if necessary, then ask a supplementary question to clarify their response:

> *'So when you took the tablets (or tried to hang yourself), you intended to die?'*

> *'So when you took the tablets, you didn't actually intend to die?'*

Triage staff should also form an initial view of the risk of harm to self by considering the patient's behaviour. Patients who are actively harming themselves and those who are threatening to harm themselves and who have the means to do so are at immediate risk (Red/priority 1) and require urgent life-saving intervention.

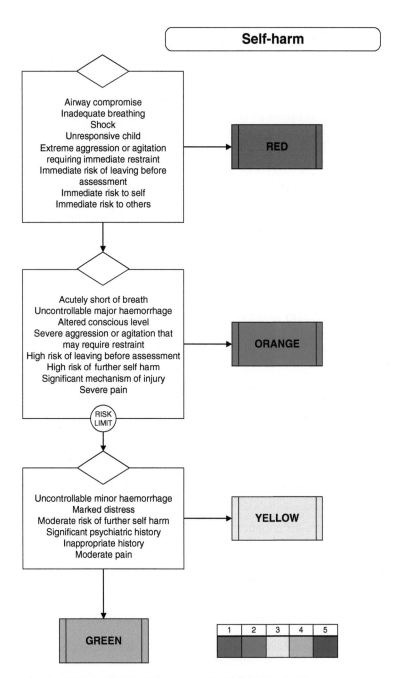

Figure 6.2 Manchester Triage System: self-harm chart
Source: Reproduced from Mackway-JonesK et al., (2013) / With permission of John Wiley & Sons.

If the patient is not deemed to be an immediate risk further questions can be asked:

'Do you have any current thoughts of harming yourself?'
'Do you have any thoughts of harming anyone else?'
'Are you okay to stay and wait in the department here until we can sort out the right help for you?'

If the patient responds to any of the questions in a way that causes concern, then the patient is at high risk (priority 2) in that they are threatening to harm themselves and are actively seeking the means to do so. In high-risk patients measures to keep them safe should be put in place. These measures will involve either arranging for a member of staff to stay with the patient or moving them to a location in the ED where they can be safely observed. The mental health team should be involved at this stage, to help with the assessment process and help form plans to keep the patient safe. Explain to the patient what you are doing and why.

'Because it was a very serious attempt (or because you still have thoughts of harming yourself) we need to keep you safe while we sort out how best to help you. We will arrange for someone to come and sit with you in the department to keep you safe.'

In most cases, close observation will not be required and the medical part of the assessment will take priority at this stage. However, if the person is identified to be at risk, a discussion should take place between the ED staff and the liaison team as to how best to integrate the physical and mental health assessments.

Likelihood of the patient leaving the ED before physical and mental health assessment can be carried out (flight risk)

Approximately 10–20% of patients who attend the ED following self-harm will leave the department before a full assessment has been completed. These patients are at higher risk of further self-harm and eventual suicide. Of most concern are those patients who walk out of an ED and go on to die by suicide within a few hours.

It is not always possible to anticipate or prevent such behaviour, but it is important to note if the patient appears restless and agitated and to alert mental health staff early if this is the case. To aid early prioritisation of these patients MTS includes discriminators to identify immediate, high and moderate levels of risk of leaving before assessment. It is helpful to explain to patients that they will be seen as quickly as possible, but they may have to wait for certain investigations to be carried out and for an assessment and help with their problems. Patients should be asked directly if they are happy with this and are willing to stay and wait. If they appear unhappy or ambivalent, discuss the situation with the mental health team, who should be available to give advice or quickly see the patient to carry out a brief risk assessment.

If a patient leaves the department before a full assessment has been done, staff should consider whether any further action is needed. If staff had concerns about that person but were not able to organise sufficient care to keep them safe, then the police must be informed as soon as possible, with a request that the person should be detained using police legal powers.

If patients have capacity to make decisions about their care, they may have a legal right to leave the ED. However, the assessment of capacity following self-harm is not straightforward and help should be sought from the mental health team, particularly if the consequences of refusal are potentially life threatening. The assessment of capacity in this situation is discussed in more detail later in this chapter. For the UK, this is described in more detail in *Guidance on Implementing the National Partnership Agreement: Right care, Right person* (NHS England, 2024) and *The Patient who Absconds* (RCEM, 2024).

Medical/surgical management

In the case of self-poisoning, methods to minimise drug absorption may need to be considered and specific toxicological advice sought from the National Poisons Centres, either by accessing TOXBASE or by telephone consultation. Specific antidotes may need to be administered, specific investigations may need to be undertaken and particular observation regimens may need to be followed.

6.5   Secondary assessment

Notwithstanding these considerations, if the patient is conscious and alert, a mental health assessment can be undertaken in parallel with physical assessment and treatment. This assessment is usually undertaken by a member of the mental health team, but such assessments can be carried out by ED staff, if suitably trained.

Mental state assessment should begin as soon as possible. When appropriate, this may be in conjunction with a physical assessment and can take place whilst blood results are awaited, or other investigations are being considered. A detailed assessment, however, can only occur if the patient is alert and fully conscious, and a period of waiting may be necessary if the patient is intoxicated. Flexible working between the ED staff and the liaison mental health team should ensure both physical and mental health assessments are completed in a timely fashion. If the patient is too intoxicated for a detailed assessment to be undertaken, the mental health team should still be available to help the ED staff manage the patient if there are concerns regarding safety and risk.

Focused conversational, compassionate, psychosocial history

> **Healthcare professionals who are empathic and compassionate encourage increased disclosure by patients about their concerns, symptoms and behaviour.**

It is best to start the mental state assessment with a brief introduction and an explanation of the purpose of the assessment, followed by an open question about the episode of self-harm:

'Could you tell me a little about what you've done?'

Try to establish the sequence of events leading up to the self-harm and what the patient actually did. How did they come to have thoughts of self-harm? What precipitated the episode? Was the self-harm planned or impulsive? Establish how they came to seek treatment in the ED.

There are many reasons why people self-harm, one of which includes a wish to end life. The most common reasons are shown in Box 6.1.

Box 6.1 Reasons why people self-harm

- Wanting to die
- Wanting to die and not wanting to die
- As a way of regulating/relieving distress
- Having time out
- To seek a reaction from others
- To express anger towards self or others
- To stop feeling isolated
- To avoid suicide

A lot of information can usually be obtained from the patient by asking relatively few questions and many of the key points you need to know may be answered naturally during the flow of the conversation. As the assessment continues, you will need to focus upon the following points if they have not already been addressed.

Assessment of risk

Identifying patients at high risk of suicide or further self-harm is an important part of most assessments following self-harm. However, in reality this is very difficult to do and most risk factors have very low predictive power.

It may be helpful to think of predicting risk as similar to trying to predict the weather. The weather forecast can be reasonably accurate over the short term (24 hours) but the longer the range, the less accurate it becomes. This is because weather is influenced by a complex, interacting pattern of meterological systems that are in constant flux. This is not so dissimilar to human behaviour, which is also subject to continual modification and change. The computer programs used to predict the weather are considerably more powerful and sophisticated than the rather crude assessments that are carried out in the ED to predict future self-harm or suicide. Therefore, any professional undertaking an assessment in an emergency situation such as the ED should focus upon the short-term risk (a few days), and be aware of the uncertainty of the clinical process. The main role of risk assessment is not to predict the future but to manage risk in the short term.

SLIPA

It is helpful to group the information gathering into five key areas (SLIPA):

SLIPA

S	Suicidal thoughts at the time of self-harm
L	**Lethality of the episode**
I	Intent now
P	Protective factors
A	**Adverse factors**

S Suicidal thoughts at the time of self-harm

This refers to the thought processes the person experienced at the time of the self-harm episode.

The patient may already have been asked about this during triage to assess any immediate risk. If so, acknowledge this:

> 'I know you may have been asked this when you first came to the emergency department this evening, but could you tell me about what was going through your mind when you. . .'

Depending upon the patient's response, you can then clarify their intent by asking:

> 'So at the time you . . . you wanted to die and intended to kill yourself?'

> 'So at the time you . . . you just wanted a break, a kind of timeout and you didn't have thoughts of actually wanting to end your life?'

Although the patient may have been asked this previously, it is important to establish it for yourself. The previous questioning will have been carried out in the context of a brief triage/screen, and the patient may have minimised their intent. The more compassionate the interview, the more likely the patient is to open up about how they are feeling and the more likely the whole assessment will be therapeutic and helpful. If the person responds that they wanted to die, establish whether they made any plans to end their life and how detailed these plans were. If the person responds that they wanted to die, sensitively but thoroughly explore this further.

Lethality of the episode

Establish the likelihood that the episode of self-harm would have resulted in death. This includes the nature of the self-harm, the steps the patient took not to be discovered and the preparation and planning involved in the episode (Box 6.2).

Box 6.2 Potential high lethality of episode of self-harm

- Violent method (e.g. hanging, gunshot, stabbing, jumping from height)
- Patient would have died without medical intervention (includes self-poisoning)
- Avoided discovery (e.g. checked into hotel, drove to a remote place, ensured they were alone)
- Made plans to kill self (e.g. bought rope, stockpiled medication)
- Anticipated death (e.g. made will or wrote a note that clearly implies patient intended to die)
- Made no active efforts to be found after the self-harm episode and did not seek help

---

Violent methods such as hanging, jumping off a high building, shooting or stabbing oneself are methods that are highly likely to result in death. Taking large amounts of medication such as paracetamol or aspirin, or taking poison, are also high-risk actions.

A degree of preparation and planning such as stockpiling medication or trying to avoid discovery by checking into a hotel or driving to an isolated location, all convey greater intent.

Find out details of the pathway to treatment. Was the person discovered by chance or did they play an active role in seeking help following the self-harm episode? In the latter case, there may still have been suicidal intent but the person changed their mind shortly after the self-harm episode, or the person may not have intended suicide and may have had some other reason for the action. Some people leave notes, which may or may not indicate suicidal intent.

 Intent now

This refers to whether the patient has any current thoughts of self-harm or suicide. This can be explored in two ways:

- Does the person have any regrets that the self-harm episode did not lead to death?
- Does the person have any current thoughts of self-harm?

  Protective and Adverse factors

Consider these two areas together as they often refer to aspects of the patient's life that can either be protective or stressful, e.g. a job can be stressful or protective or both. Common aspects are personal relationships, family and friends, job, housing, finances and criminal charges.

Approximately 70% of all self-harm episodes are precipitated by some kind of interpersonal problem, e.g. marriage break up, bereavement, domestic abuse, miscarriage or argument. So always enquire about this aspect of the patient's life and find out about their living circumstances. Are they living alone, or if they are living with someone, is this a supportive relationship?

Thoughts of hopelessness can be a significant adverse factor.

Establish how able they are to resist any suicidal thoughts and how easy it is for them to access their intended method of self-harm/suicide.

Assessment of these five SLIPA areas provides the basis for the assessment of risk to which other relevant factors can be added to produce an overall risk profile. As stated earlier this is not an exact science and advice from a more experienced professional should be sought if there are concerns or doubts about the process. Some examples of how a risk profile is constructed are given later in this chapter.

Demographic or historical risk factors

Known risk factors are listed in Box 6.3. Individually these factors have low predictive power as they have been identified from large longitudinal cohort studies, in which basic information recorded in patients' notes has been used to predict later suicide. Such studies rarely include detailed information obtained by assessing people's actual mental states at the time of the self-harm episode. We suggest that the demographic/historical risk factors should be combined with the information obtained from SLIPA to enhance the accuracy of the risk assessment. Many patients who present with self-harm

---

Box 6.3 Demographic or historical risk factors for suicide

- Male
- Middle or older age
- Living alone
- Previous history of self-harm
- Previous history of severe mental illness (includes schizophrenia, bipolar disorder and depression)
- History of drug dependence
- History of violent behaviour
- Frequent ED attendances
- Alcohol problems
- Unemployed
- Socially isolated
- Severe or long-term physical illness
- Significant date (e.g. anniversary of loss of a loved one)
- Homelessness

have at least one or two or more of these demographic/historical factors (e.g. male and unemployed), so it is difficult to make clinical judgements based upon these factors alone.

Co-morbid mental illness

Self-harm is not a psychiatric diagnosis in itself. It is a behaviour which signals that an individual is not able to cope with a particular situation or set of circumstances. Self-harm is often associated with mental illness, as mental illness often impairs an individual's ability to cope. Approximately 70% of patients who self-harm have a co-morbid mental illness, and mental illness is a strong risk factor for suicide. Often there is a pattern of symptoms worsening or building up, which lead to the self-harm episode.

Appropriate treatment of any co-morbid conditions may reduce the risk of future self-harm or suicide. Patients with severe mental illness, either schizophrenia or bipolar affective disorder, who have self-harmed must have a detailed assessment from a mental health professional to ensure an appropriate treatment and management plan is put in place.

The most common co-morbid problems associated with self-harm are depression or substance misuse. Key symptoms for depression include persistent low mood for at least 2 weeks or longer, poor sleep, poor appetite, weight loss, poor concentration, morbid thoughts, inability to enjoy things, low energy and drive, irritability, fatigue, guilt or a feeling that life is not worth living. Box 6.4 lists all of the most common symptoms of depression. Feelings of hopelessness have been linked to an increased risk of suicide and should always be enquired about.

Box 6.4 Common symptoms of depression

Mood symptoms
- Persistent low mood
- Diurnal variation in mood (typically worse in the morning)
- Anhedonia – being unable to enjoy things

Physical symptoms
- Poor sleep – early morning wakening or repeated waking throughout the night or difficulty getting off to sleep
- Poor appetite
- Weight loss
- Lack of energy

Cognitive symptoms
- Guilt
- Hopelessness
- Belief that life is not worth living
- Suicidal ideation
- Feeling a burden on others
- Poor concentration
- Forgetfulness

Alcohol and drug problems

Many episodes of self-harm occur in the context of taking alcohol or drugs. This may indicate an underlying problem with alcohol or drugs, which will increase the likelihood of further episodes of self-harm if the problem is not addressed. Try to ascertain how much alcohol or drugs the patient took prior to the self-harm and whether this made a significant contribution to the self-harm act. Does the patient recognise the contribution that alcohol or drugs made, and want help to cut down or abstain?

Try to establish how much alcohol the patient consumes on a weekly basis, and the amount of illicit drugs the patient takes. Screen for any evidence of alcohol dependence, particularly if the patient is likely to be admitted, as they will need to be started on an appropriate withdrawal and vitamin replacement regime by the admitting team. The management of patients with alcohol and drug-related problems is covered in detail in Chapter 8.

Co-morbid physical health problems

The risk of suicide is significantly elevated in patients with severe physical illness. Screen for any physical health problems, particularly those associated with excessive alcohol consumption; including a history of fits, liver problems, neurological problems or gastrointestinal disorders. Have a high index of suspicion for patients who self-harm in the context of terminal illness. Although an individual may come to a careful and thoughtful decision to end their life in the context of a terminal illness, a sudden or impulsive action is unlikely to have been thought through and often indicates the patient is struggling to come to terms with the illness, or may have become depressed.

Developing a risk profile

Start with the information from SLIPA and use additional relevant information to build the profile, as in Figure 6.3. This will include taking account of demographic and historical factors, and the presence or absence of mental illness. The information from SLIPA should carry the most weight, as it is most directly related to managing current risk, with 'co-morbid mental illness' also important. The demographic and historical factors should be used as adjuncts but **not** as stand-alone measures.

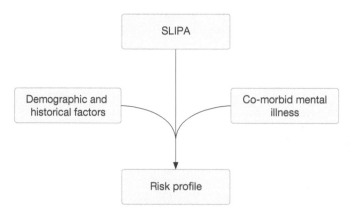

Figure 6.3 Building a risk profile in self-harm

6.6   Emergency management

If the patient requires admission to the acute hospital for either monitoring of cardiac status or requires further treatment, a clear initial plan for managing psychiatric aspects of care should be written in the notes and conveyed to the staff who will take over the medical care. As a priority this must include the level of observation required over the next 24–48 hours (Box 6.5).

Box 6.5 Potential levels of observation

- No additional observation
- No specific observation but should not be allowed to leave without full mental health assessment. If necessary in an emergency situation, use legal powers to hold the patient on a mental health ward in order for an assessment to be arranged (provided the patient has been formally admitted to hospital)
- Close observation required (every 15 minutes)
- One-to-one observation required (preferably by a mental health trained nurse)
- More than one-to-one observation. Risk requires more than one member of staff (preferably by mental health trained nurses)

The plan must state when the patient should be reviewed by a member of the mental health liaison team, for example when conscious and alert, or if staff have concerns about the patient's mental health or behaviour.

The plan should also include advice regarding psychotropic medication. If the patient is known to services and the regular medication they take can be established, then this should be continued unless there are medical contraindications. This is particularly important in the case of clozapine: if the treatment is interrupted for more than 48 hours, the drug has to be restarted from baseline and titrated slowly up to therapeutic dosage, which can take several weeks.

If the patient is medically fit and does not require psychiatric admission or treatment from the crisis or home treatment team, a clear management plan must be developed and agreed with the patient. This will include advice about further treatment and referral to or follow-up by other services. It should also include advice about seeking help in a crisis situation with telephone help lines and contact numbers of crisis services. Patients should receive a leaflet summarising this advice and information. It is also good practice to ask whether the patient has a Safety Plan and, if not, to help them develop one. A Safety Plan is a structured, proactive way to help people plan and arrange a series of activities and sources of support that they can activate if they begin to have suicidal thoughts.

The Royal College of Psychiatrists recommends the Stay Alive suicide prevention app (http://prevent-suicide.org.uk/stay_alive_suicide_prevention_mobile_phone_application.html) and the distrACT app for self-harm (http://www.expertselfcare.com/health-apps/distract/).

Stayingsafe.net is a great resource to direct patients to. There are videos and advice to aid them making a Safety Plan.

Patients may be offered brief psychological treatment following self-harm by a specialist self-harm team and will be contacted the following day by the team. Wherever possible, arrangements should be made for the patient to return home with a partner, family member or friend and for someone to be with them over the next 24–48 hours. It is important to discuss with the patient and a family member/friend (if possible) the removal of any tablets that could be used for further self-harm, or if the person has any razor blades, etc. that these too could be removed.

If the patient is medically fit and requires either admission to an in-patient psychiatric unit or crisis team input, this will be organised by the mental health liaison team. Advice about observation regimes and routine medication should be clearly recorded and discussed with the accepting team members (either ward or crisis team). The patient's physical health needs and physical health medications should also be recorded and this information should be discussed fully with the accepting team.

6.7 Refusal to accept physical treatment following self-harm

Some patients attend the ED following self-harm but then refuse the physical investigations or physical treatment that is necessary either to save life or treat the physical consequences of the self-harm.

This can be a difficult and somewhat frustrating scenario for staff, who may not feel they have time to negotiate or persuade someone to have treatment whilst other patients in the department are waiting and, in some cases, urgently need care.

Staff, however, have a duty of care to all patients and must try to offer appropriate help and treatment. The refusal is often linked to a continued desire to die or, more commonly, to deeper psychological difficulties or problems the patient has with caring or being cared for.

Whatever the reason, clear guidance about what to do in such a scenario often relieves staff anxiety.

Firstly, most patients, given some time and the ability to talk about their problems, will consent to treatment. A calm, sympathetic and compassionate approach by staff, and a willingness to try to understand the reasons why the patient is refusing treatment, usually results in a resolution of the situation. The use of written information about any treatment that is being proposed can help improve understanding and retention of information, and enable the person to think through the options.

Secondly, if the person continues to refuse, NICE has developed guidelines (NG225, 2022) laying out how to manage the situation. These are principally determined by a judgement that staff make about the person's capacity to make a potentially life-threatening decision regarding their care.

Capacity in self-harm

In England and Wales, the law states that patients have the right to refuse treatment for their health even if it might seem unwise, if they have capacity to do so. Capacity is presumed, but in the case of someone refusing life-saving treatment, capacity must be assessed. This section refers specifically to issues concerning the assessment of capacity following refusal for treatment after a person has self-harmed. It is presumed that the self-harm under consideration is potentially life threatening, and refusal of the treatment would result in either serious physical harm or death.

It is possible for people who are suffering from severe mental illness to make capacitous decisions about certain aspects of their medical care or treatment, and there is case law to support this. The mental disturbance, however, must not impair the decision-making process regarding the treatment decision in question. Mental capacity assessment has a two-stage test. First, a person must not be suffering from a disturbance of mind. Second, they must be able to:

1. Understand information given to them about treatment options and the necessity for treatment
2. Retain information relevant to the treatment options
3. Use or weigh that information in coming to a decision
4. Communicate that decision

A patient who is delirious or severely intoxicated from either drugs or alcohol is likely to be unable to either understand or retain information, and this is usually fairly straightforward for most staff to determine.

In cases where the patient is conscious, alert and fully orientated, a common mistake is to ask the patient some brief questions about the self-harm episode and the person's wishes and assume from that brief contact that the patient has capacity. In this scenario, the patient probably meets the first two criteria for capacity (can understand and retain information). However, the third criteria (whether the person can weigh up the decision they need to make) is the key issue. This can be affected by serious emotional turmoil (depression, anxiety, loss, despair) and other forms of mental illness, and has been shown to have more impact in psychiatric in-patients than medical in-patients.

As an example, when people become depressed, the way they view the world, and themselves, changes. As part of their depressive disorder, they may develop negative thoughts which can be wide ranging and may include ideas about being worthless, or being a bad person, or feeling hopeless or guilty and that life is not worth living. These thought processes are regarded by psychiatrists as symptoms of an illness, which will change with treatment. However, a person with these symptoms, if questioned by an ED member of staff, may well say that they do not want treatment and want to die. This may then be accepted at face value as a capacitous decision, whereas the person is actually suffering from a mental illness that is impairing their decision-making abilities. High emotional arousal or distress, both of which are common in self-harm, can also affect decision making.

Even if the patient does not appear grossly intoxicated, the presence of drugs or alcohol in their blood may have an effect upon decision making.

In the emergency setting, the ability to weigh up a decision can be extremely difficult. Clinicians are advised to have a low threshold for asking for advice or a second opinion (Box 6.6).

Box 6.6 Assessment of mental capacity in a person refusing life-saving treatment following self-harm

Explain the treatment that is required, what it entails and why it is necessary. If possible provide written information.

- Can the person understand the information?
- Can the person retain the information you have given them?

NB: Patients who are delirious or are severely intoxicated are very unlikely to meet these first two criteria.

- Try to establish whether the person can weigh in the balance their refusal to have treatment:

1. Ask why the person is refusing to have the treatment
2. Check they understand the likely physical consequences of refusing the treatment (i.e. death or serious physical sequelae)
3. Ask the person to describe to you how they have come to this decision and what things they have considered
4. Ask the person about how they have been feeling recently. Specifically ask if they have been feeling fed up or low, anxious or stressed
5. Ask about contact with mental health services or psychotropic medication such as antidepressants
6. Ask about recent contact with the GP for stress or depression
7. Assess if they have recently consumed drugs or alcohol in the last 24 hours

IF YES TO ANY OF THE ABOVE CONSIDER REQUESTING A PSYCHIATRIC OPINION

- If the person's responses to questions 1 to 7 lead you to believe their decision making is impaired, and urgent treatment is required to save life or serious physical harm, start treatment in their best interests before psychiatric assessment

---

If the patient is deemed not to have capacity to consent to treatment, then staff must act in the person's best interests. In non-emergency scenarios, this would involve a 'best interests' meeting with all relevant health professionals and the patient's family or representatives in attendance. In the emergency situation, staff should act to save life or prevent irremediable harm as this is considered to be the most likely action to be in the patient's best interests.

This may involve sedation, if the patient continues to refuse treatment, so that the necessary medical intervention can be implemented. In most cases, however, the person usually agrees to treatment being implemented if the situation is explained carefully to them by staff.

The role of legal frameworks

If a patient has seriously self-harmed (e.g. tried to hang themselves or has taken a very significant overdose), and they are attempting to leave the department, there are likely to be grounds to detain them under mental health laws for further assessment of their mental condition.

In the setting of an acute medical ward or short stay unit, consent from a patient detained under the Mental Health Act will not be required for any **medical** treatment given to them for the mental disorder from which they are suffering, although medical treatment of an unrelated physical condition would not be allowed. Medical treatment may include nasogastric feeding in anorexia nervosa, and although it has not been tested in the courts, it is likely to include life-saving treatment following self-harm.

Advance decisions

Advance decisions (also known as advanced directives or advanced statements depending on jurisdiction) are prospectively written statements that may be legally binding in some countries. They make provision for individuals to determine the kind of treatment (or no treatment) that they would like to receive in the event they become ill and incapacitous. Individuals need to be capacitous at the time they make the advance decision. Refusals of life-saving treatment must be expressed in writing, witnessed and include a statement that the decision stands even if life is at risk.

Advance decisions are a very difficult area. If staff are in any doubt, they should consult a senior psychiatrist as an advance decision does not preclude the use of legal powers if there are grounds to use them. Legal advice can also often be obtained by NHS Trusts or Boards very quickly in an emergency situation.

High impact users (previously known as multiple or frequent attenders) attending with self-harm

Some individuals present on multiple occasions with self-harm. This may be to the same ED or to several departments in a similar geographical area, or to EDs all over the country. The self-harm behaviour often has low risk of lethality, although this is not always the case, and the self-harming is often associated with drug or alcohol abuse, unemployment, poor social circumstances and homelessness.

Frequent attendance for self-harm is associated with a higher risk of suicide and early death following attendance. A history of alcohol abuse and unemployment are also important contributory factors.

The attendance of a patient on three or more occasions within a 12-month period to the ED with self-harm or requests for psychiatric help should trigger a review of care. This will require a coordinated approach between the ED and community and mental health services. If the person is under mental health services, a care plan should already have been drawn up, which should be reviewed in light of the new episodes of self-harm or ED attendances. This plan ideally should have involved the patient. If the person is not under the care of mental health services, they should be offered the option of follow-up and further assessment from either primary care or secondary care mental health teams. The GP and all other relevant health professionals should be fully involved and informed of these actions. Clinicians should be alert to the possible association of an increased frequency of attendance at the ED and suicide.

Although many of these people have complex psychosocial problems, increased frequency of attendance is often triggered by a recent current stressor. If the person receives help for this, it can reduce ED attendance and the risk of suicide in the short term, even if the underlying problems are very longstanding.

6.8   Case examples

The following cases show how to develop a psychiatric risk profile. This sits in the secondary assessment. Primary assessment is not illustrated in these cases. Any medical issues highlighted in these cases are being concurrently managed.

Case 6.1

A 42-year-old Polish man, Aleksander, jumped 40 feet from scaffolding, resulting in multiple fractures to his back and pelvis. His right lower leg had to be amputated at the scene as it became trapped in the scaffolding on his way down. Aleksander has worked as a labourer but has been unable to find work for several months prior to the episode, and is about to be evicted from his flat. He is estranged from his wife who is preventing him from having access to his 9-year-old daughter, whom he has been unable to see for several months. He has been low in mood for several weeks prior to the self-harm episode. He intended to die.

SLIPA	**S**uicidal thoughts at time of episode: yes **L**ethality: very high **I**ntent now: no current intent when assessed in hospital **P**rotective factors: none identified **A**dverse factors: inability to find work, low income, homelessness; lack of access to daughter; social isolation; amputation of leg will impair likelihood of being able to work again as a labourer in the future
Demographic and historical factors	Male Middle aged Homeless Social isolation Unemployed
Co-morbid mental illness	Evidence of a depressive illness developing in the weeks prior to the self-harm episode. No alcohol or drug misuse
Risk profile	The overall risk profile in this case is high as most of the SLIPA items are positive; the patient also has four demographic/historical risk factors and in addition is suffering from a depressive illness The patient requires immediate treatment for his physical injuries and fractures with admission to an orthopaedic ward. He may require close observation (one-to-one) on the orthopaedic ward by clinical staff. Ongoing psychiatric liaison team management will be required. A full mental health assessment will be required

Case 6.2

A 29-year-old woman, Aoife, took an overdose of antidepressants which she has been prescribed by her GP. She has been under increasing pressure at work and has felt low in mood and panicky for the last 3 months. She is constantly tired but can't sleep well and has lost 4 kg in weight. She has begun to drink a bottle of wine per night to help with the panicky feelings and her sleep. Her husband is in the armed forces and has been away on a tour of duty for several months. She had a miscarriage in the previous year, which she has found very difficult to come to terms with. She took the tablets (20 mirtazapine 15 mg tablets) late at night after she had been drinking heavily. She did not take them because she wanted to die, but rather because she wanted to sleep. She panicked after taking them and immediately phoned a friend who brought her to the hospital.

SLIPA	**S**uicidal thoughts at time of episode: no **L**ethality: low **I**ntent now: no current intent when assessed in hospital **P**rotective factors: working, married, has good friend **A**dverse factors: work is stressful, husband is away, recent miscarriage, alcohol misuse
Demographic or historical factors	Alcohol and depression
Co-morbid mental illness	Evidence of a depressive illness developing in the weeks prior to the self-harm episode. Excess alcohol intake and self-harm episode took place in context of heavy drinking that evening
Risk profile	The overall risk profile in this case is probably low as most of the SLIPA items are negative and the patient has no identified demographic/historical risk factors other than alcohol consumption. The patient has developed a depressive illness, which has not responded to antidepressants and appears to have been precipitated by a variety of interpersonal difficulties The patient requires help for her depression, which will include an alternative antidepressant (with advice from her GP to prescribe only a maximum of 1 week's supply at a time) plus psychological treatment. She has agreed to engage with alcohol services. Her GP will be asked to monitor her over the next few weeks

Case 6.3

Leah, a 23-year-old woman, is brought to the ED after she tried to hang herself. She had taken ketamine with some friends at a party. She became very distressed after taking the drug and used a belt to try to hang herself in the toilet. Two friends found her and cut her down. She was alert when being assessed in the ED but has a superficial mark to her throat from the belt. She has very little memory of the incident or why she tried to kill herself. She has a prior history of taking an overdose when she was 16 years old, after the break up of a relationship, but otherwise has been well and had not been in contact with mental services. She is doing a PhD at the local university. She has a supportive circle of friends, and a boyfriend of 2 years. All her friends use recreational drugs.

SLIPA	**S**uicidal thoughts at time of episode: unknown **L**ethality: high **I**ntent now: no current intent when assessed in hospital **P**rotective factors: PhD course, friends, boyfriend **A**dverse factors: all her friends use recreational drugs which may make it difficult for her to abstain in the future
Demographic or historical factors	None identified
Co-morbid mental illness	Uses recreational drugs, mainly ketamine, at weekends
Risk profile	The risk profile for this patient is uncertain. It is probably moderate as there is a mixed response to the SLIPA items; the episode itself had high lethality, although it did not appear to have been planned There are demographic and historical risk factors. The patient uses recreational drugs, which appear to be the precipitant of the self-harm episode. However, there is no evidence of current depressive illness Her mental state at the time of the attempted self-harm was unknown; she will require close follow-up to establish ongoing risk

6.9 Summary

Presentations of people who self-harm are common in the ED. These people should receive integrated physical and mental healthcare, with timely assessment and treatment. People who are at high risk of imminent further self-harm should be identified at an early stage and appropriate measures put in place to keep them safe whilst physical and mental health assessments are carried out. People who self-harm should be involved as much as possible in decisions about their care.

Those people who have self-harmed and wish to leave the ED, before a full assessment can be completed, require an assessment of their capacity. If there is concern that their decision-making skills are impaired due to their psychological state, a psychiatric opinion should be sought. If they are deemed to be capacitous, their wishes should be respected and they should be allowed to leave.

ED staff should feel confident in their management of both the physical and basic mental health components of care, and work collaboratively with the liaison psychiatry team to provide high-quality, person-centred care.

CHAPTER 7

Organic causes for behavioural disturbances

Learning outcomes

After reading this chapter, you will be able to:

- Identify how to rapidly and systematically assess the patient presenting with an apparent mental health emergency or apparent intoxication
- Characterise common co-morbid problems and mimics of psychiatric presentations
- Demonstrate how to work through common, urgent psychiatric scenarios that can present as a medical problem

---

7.1 Introduction

This chapter will look at when to consider alternative diagnoses in a patient attending with an apparent mental health emergency or apparent intoxication – the 'wolf in sheep's clothing'. It is also necessary to be aware of diagnostic overshadowing – either underplaying medical symptoms or attributing them to previous mental health conditions. Having a mental health disorder impacts on physical health, increasing the impact of chronic diseases such as chronic obstructive pulmonary disease, heart disease and diabetes. Mental health disorders are also associated with drug and alcohol misuse, either as part of the cause or as part of an attempt at self-management of symptoms.

Acute Psychiatric Emergencies: A Practical Approach, Second Edition.
Edited by Mark Buchanan and Damien Longson.
© 2025 John Wiley & Sons Ltd. Published 2025 by John Wiley & Sons Ltd.

7.2   Is there a likely medical issue?

The focus here is achieving diagnostic clarity and contingency planning to manage any potential medical or surgical condition. A psychiatric ward is not an appropriate environment for a patient with an acute non-psychiatric condition.

It is important to acknowledge that there are medical presentations that can present alongside or indeed masquerade as a psychiatric presentation.

However, unnecessary investigations may delay appropriate management of the mental health emergency. This delay is against National Institute for Health and Care Excellence (NICE) self-harm guidance and the *Side by Side* document signed up to by the Royal College of Psychiatrists (RCPsych), Royal College of Emergency Medicine (RCEM), Royal College of Physicians (RCP) and Royal College of Nursing (RCN).

There are certain situations that increase the risk that there may be a medical issue that needs attending to. These include extremes of age, new-onset psychiatric presentation, abnormal vital sign observations, certain co-morbidities, medications, overdose/self-harm or evidence of trauma. Possible intoxication/withdrawal is also important to consider, and this is expanded on later in this chapter. The SMART Form (Figure 7.1) is a useful tool created by the Sierra Sacramento Valley Medical Society to reduce delays in access for patients in EDs accessing psychiatric input.

SMART

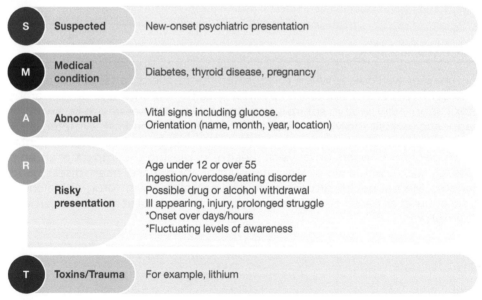

S	Suspected	New-onset psychiatric presentation
M	Medical condition	Diabetes, thyroid disease, pregnancy
A	Abnormal	Vital signs including glucose. Orientation (name, month, year, location)
R	Risky presentation	Age under 12 or over 55 Ingestion/overdose/eating disorder Possible drug or alcohol withdrawal Ill appearing, injury, prolonged struggle *Onset over days/hours *Fluctuating levels of awareness
T	Toxins/Trauma	For example, lithium

* Not in the original form but seen as a risky presentation

Figure 7.1 SMART Form
Source: Adapted from Sierra Sacramento Valley Medical Society: smart medicalclearance.org

If the answer is no to each part of the tool, the likelihood of a medical cause is low, reducing the need for medical tests. History and physical examination alone detect up to 95% of abnormalities (Olshaker et al., 1997).

New-onset psychiatric presentations are associated with a high possibility of an organic cause and so should prompt the need for a more in-depth medical assessment. Side-by-side assessment with the mental health team is still required.

The presence of abnormal physical signs or disorientation are the most obvious flags that there may be an organic cause.

7.3 Secondary assessment

After immediate, life-threatening injuries and serious risks have been either excluded or addressed, the parallel assessment should proceed towards arriving at a working diagnosis with plans for treating urgent physical and mental health problems.

Focused physical history and secondary examination

Gather any collateral information from nurses, paramedics, police or accompanying others (such as where and when was the patient found, key concerns at the scene including injuries, seizures, persistent vomiting, initial Glasgow Coma Scale (GCS) score and physical observations, aggression, suicidality and self-harm or hallucinations). Is the patient being held under legal powers, and why?

There should be a brief review of the latest observations, GCS score and medication chart (blood tests and electrocardiogram (ECG) if readily available and if appropriate).

Focused history: PHRASED

The PHRASED focused history (see Figure 3.3) can be adapted in the following ways to ensure that mental health issues are considered.

(P) *Presenting complaint*

(H) *History of presenting complaint*

Is there any suspicion here of self-harm? If so, proceed to the SLIPA risk assessment.

(R) *Relevant medical history*

Past and recent medical and psychiatric history, and knowledge of what medications the patient is taking, is important. This may aid the diagnosis of the patient's current problem. Lists of medications and medical diagnoses that can cause mental health symptoms and conditions are given later in this chapter.

Ask about:

- Disorders associated with psychosis such as schizophrenia and schizoaffective disorder, depression and bipolar affective disorder
- Conditions associated with chronic cognitive impairment such as learning difficulties, dementias and acquired brain injury

(A) *Allergies*

(S) *Systems review*

(E) *Essential family and social history*

Include:

- Age
- First language
- History of self-harm or violence towards others
- Forensic history – particularly violence towards others and damage to property

(D) *Drugs (medication and drugs of misuse)*

See the patient's past medical history in relation to medication and drugs. Take a drug and alcohol history. If substances have been consumed, quantify the amount and type, the timeframe (all at once, over several hours, etc.) and whether this amount is typical for the patient.

Secondary examination/investigations: guided by focused history

Think SMART.

- Top-to-toe physical examination (including neurological examination – this is essential)
- Investigations – as directed by history or examination findings

If after this assessment the patient does not have any indicators for an organic cause, it is more likely to be a primary psychiatric presentation. If there are new or ongoing concerns, then these should be addressed.

7.4 Management of specific clinical presentations

Overdose

If overdose is suspected, anticipate the medical complications of the drug. In the UK, TOXBASE is a helpful resource that gives information about the investigation and management of the drug taken.

Alcohol (see Chapter 8)

If there is any suspicion of alcohol misuse, always give thiamine. Do not wait hours to see if this situation resolves.

Suicidality and attempted self-harm (see Chapter 6)

Depressed mood, suicidal thoughts and attempted self-harm are common co-morbid features of alcohol-associated presentations to the ED. Assessment of self-harm is covered in detail elsewhere, but specific aspects of assessment in the patient presenting with intoxication are given here.

Establish the severity of depression and associated risks. If the patient has ongoing suicidal thoughts and they are thinking of, or have recently acted on, these thoughts they should be under one-to-one observation.

- Do suicidal thoughts intensify when intoxicated?
- Have these thoughts ever led to self-harm – was the patient intoxicated at the time and was self-harm planned, impulsive or accidental?
- Does the patient have any concern for their own safety when intoxicated (could provide a window of opportunity for intervention)?
- Is there a temporal relationship between the development of depressed mood/anxiety and alcohol misuse?
- Try to establish which came first. Is there a history of significant life events that precipitated either low mood or alcohol misuse?
- Does alcohol help to blot out difficult feelings and memories, quell anxiety or aid sleep?
- Are mood, appetite and energy levels better when abstinent from alcohol?

Psychotic symptoms (see Chapter 9)

Ascertain the severity and range of symptoms and any associated risks to the patient or others. Ask about content of hallucinations and whether the patient has any concerns about being watched, spied on or being harmed or whether they have any concerns about their partner. Morbid jealousy is a recognised complication of chronic, heavy alcohol use and delusions of infidelity can confer significant risk to the patient's partner and the suspected seducer. Try to establish whether there is an association between heavy drinking and the development or worsening of symptoms or whether the patient has recently become abstinent. Is there a previous history of schizophrenia, schizoaffective disorder, mood disorder with psychosis, drug-induced psychosis (culprit drug?), alcoholic hallucinosis (worsens with heavy drinking) or delirium tremens? If there is a history of a psychotic disorder, try to establish whether the patient is compliant with their medication regime, whether they find it effective or whether they sometimes use alcohol to reduce the impact of distressing hallucinations and delusional beliefs.

Significantly confused (see Chapter 9)

Is there any history of cognitive impairment? If unable to sit through a formal test such as the MoCA (Montreal Cognitive Assessment), check whether the patient is orientated, can name months of the year backwards and can recall five words immediately (e.g. apple, table, yellow, church, rose) and after a 5-minute delay. If confusion is due to alcohol intoxication it should begin to improve within a few hours of abstinence. Consider the presence of Wernicke's encephalopathy. Check eye movements (lateral movements are often impaired due to VI nerve palsy, and nystagmus may also be present), gait (broad based and unsteady) and truncal stability (may be difficult to remain sitting upright without support). This requires immediate treatment with thiamine. Cognitive tests should be repeated in a few hours to check for any changes. If confusion is not resolving, discuss with the ED team and review examination and investigation results so that further options can be explored.

7.5   Emergency management: principles of shared care

Teams should share the following perspectives if they have assessed in parallel:

- **Physical health team:** Is there any evidence of physical health problems or toxic/withdrawal states that could explain or be contributing to the current presentation? If so, what is the working diagnosis and plan for further investigations and treatment? Were any mental health concerns picked up during assessment that should be discussed with the mental health team?
- **Mental health team:** Have acute mental health concerns been identified and if so how should they be monitored and managed? Are there immediate and ongoing risks to self and others? What is the immediate plan for managing these? Is there a suspicion of co-ingestion of other substances? Were any physical health concerns picked up during assessment that should be discussed with the ED team?
- **Both teams:** Has the patient's capacity to consent to or refuse to remain in hospital to have further investigations and treatment been established? If an extremely agitated, unwell patient is refusing further input and lacks capacity, an urgent joint plan must be implemented that enables action in the patient's best interests. This may involve rapid tranquillisation to reduce distress and agitation and to enable further investigation and treatment.

7.6   Determine outcomes and ongoing care plan

1. Significant injuries and/or other physical health problems warrant in-patient admission with the patient remaining in a general hospital setting for further investigations and treatment. If mental health problems were also identified, ongoing input from the liaison mental health team is needed to review progress, and to advise on managing risks and discharge planning.
2. Where routine physical examination and investigations are normal but severe and acute mental health problems have been identified that confer risks to patient and others, the mental health team should determine whether admission to a psychiatry in-patient unit or discharge with intensive support from crisis services in the community is appropriate.
3. If an individual is significantly abusive and aggressive but no discernible physical or mental health problems beyond alcohol misuse were identified by the assessing teams, perspectives should be shared. Joint agreement should be reached on requesting assistance from hospital security and the police to remove the individual from the department and discussing whether assault or criminal damage charges are appropriate.

7.7   Organic disorders with psychiatric presentations

Insidious onset

In some inherited neurological conditions, psychiatric symptoms may be the first presenting sign. Often the onset is insidious over many years and may include significant change in personality. Many of these disorders can lead to delirium as well as specific psychiatric symptoms.

Acromegaly – depression, irritability, apathy or labile mood
Acute confusional state and dementia – see Chapter 9
Addison's disease – depression, anxiety and irritability
Cerebral tumours – depression or emotional lability. Symptoms may depend on the location of the tumour: occipital may cause visual hallucinations; temporal lobe may cause visual and auditory hallucinations; parietal tumours are associated with tactile and kinaesthetic hallucinations; frontal tumours may cause disinhibition and a variety of hallucinations; diencephalic tumours may present as Korsakoff's psychosis
Cerebrovascular disorders – delirium, organic psychoses, mood disorders and personality change
Charles Bonnet syndrome – ocular pathology is related to visual hallucinations which are often complex and vivid and tend to occur at times of low light. The patient often has full insight and is undistressed
Cushing's syndrome – depression, mania and psychosis
Head injury – organic schizophrenia and affective psychoses. Personality change

HIV (human immunodeficiency virus) – dementia

Huntington's chorea – may present with depression, aggression, psychosis or obsessive compulsive disorder

Hyperparathyroidism – depression

Hyperprolactinaemia – severe depression

Hyperthyroidism – hypomania/mania, psychosis and anxiety

Hypoparathyroidism – may rarely present with psychoses

Hypopituitarism – depression often with irritability and features of dementia

Hypothyroidism – severe depression with or without psychotic symptoms, may present as early dementia

Inherited leucodystrophies (metachromatic leucodystrophy) – psychotic symptoms

Motor neurone disease – emotional lability

Multiple sclerosis – depression, mania and psychosis

Neuroacanthocytosis – depression, anxiety, obsessive compulsive disorder and personality change

Paraneoplastic syndrome – psychoses and affective symptoms

Parkinson's disease – depression

Peduncular hallucinosis – damage to the midbrain/thalamus causes vivid visual hallucinations, often in the evenings

Pellagra – delirium, depression and psychoses

Phaeochromocytoma – chronic anxiety and panic disorder

Polyarteritis nodosa – delirium, mania and paranoia

Spinocerebellar ataxia – personality change, labile mood, aggression or dysexecutive syndrome

Sporadic Creutzfeldt–Jakob disease – rapidly progressive dementia

Syphilis – may present in a variety of ways including dementia, depression and elation or with schizophrenic features

Systemic lupus erythematosus – psychotic symptoms

Variant Creutzfeldt–Jakob disease – depression or anxiety

Wilson's disease – personality change, mood disturbance, psychosis and cognitive impairment

Acute onset

Acute intermittent porphyria – psychotic symptoms

Carbon monoxide poisoning – may present as Korsakoff's psychosis

Encephalitis (including anti-N-methyl-D-aspartate receptor and anti-voltage-gated potassium channel antibody-associated limbic encephalitis) – psychotic symptoms and delirium

Epilepsy:
- Temporal lobe epilepsy – hallucinations in all modalities, may appear to have thought blocking, déjà vu, jamais vu and affective symptoms
- Per-ictal, inter-ictal and post-ictal psychosis
- Complex partial seizure – may lead to epileptic automatism (the patient may perform often simple but at times complex activities while suffering from reduced consciousness)

- Fugue – patients may appear drowsy or intoxicated, and often undertake complex behaviours and wander large distances, waking in an unknown area with no idea how they arrived there. These states may last from hours to rarely weeks at a time
- Parietal and occipital lesions – may cause visual phenomena
- Transient global amnesia

Head injury – may cause aggressive behaviour, agitation, amnesia and confusional states

Hepatic encephalopathy – delirium

Migraine – depression, anxiety, irritability and complex auditory and visual hallucinations

7.8 Medications and psychiatric side effects

Prescribed and over-the-counter medications can have psychiatric side effects even in normal doses. The list in Table 7.1 is not exhaustive.

Table 7.1 Psychiatric side effects of common medications	
Medication type	**Commonly associated side effects**
Antiepileptics	Delirium, psychosis, irritability
Steroids (corticosteroids and anabolic)	Mood changes
Fluoroquinolones	Restlessness, irritability
Aciclovir/ganciclovir	Hallucinations
Dopaminergic, e.g. anti-Parkinson agents	Psychosis, agitation, irritability
Anticholinergics	Delirium
Beta-blockers	Delirium, psychosis, depression

7.9 Handover

Risks should be reassessed, and essential information regarding presentation, working diagnosis and treatment plan, should be collated for handover to the receiving team using SBAR (see Chapter 13).

7.10 Case examples

Case 7.1

Tetsuya, a 57-year-old man, is brought into the ED by the police. Local train station staff contacted the police after members of the public expressed concerns that a man was locked in a toilet cubicle, muttering to himself. Since arrival in the department, he has been very anxious. It is difficult to follow his conversation, but he seems to be talking about being followed and appears to be very wary of the accompanying police officers and is constantly asking passing staff to help keep him safe. Looks appropriately dressed but is carrying a plastic bag, which he is unwilling to put down. The police officers had searched the bag, which contains paperwork including his passport.

Primary assessment	ABCD	**A** – Maintaining own airway **B** – RR 18, SpO_2 98% **C** – HR 86 bpm, BP 135/85 **D** – Alert, PERLA, glucose 5.5 mmol/L	AEIO	**A** – Anxious and aroused, with possible delusional thoughts **E** – Transferred to safe room from triage. Police present **I** – No obvious risk to self or others. Moderate to high risk of leaving due to irrational thoughts **O** – No dangerous objects
SMART		**S**MART assessment – positive **S**uspected new onset (patient not known to your area) **R**isky presentation – over 55		
Unified assessment and immediate treatment		No immediate physical risk identified; no immediate mental health treatment required and, currently, need for rapid tranquillisation is low. Containment plan to include discrete one-to-one security presence		
Secondary assessment				
Focused physical history and secondary examination		A PHRASED physical history reveals no physical complaints, except for mild hypertension (admits recent non-compliance with his antihypertensives as he has been too worried to pick up his prescription) Physical examination is unremarkable, as are routine bloods and ECG		

Focused conversational psychosocial history and mental state examination (MSE)	Tetsuya believes that government agents are following him using cars, as well as spying on him with security cameras and electronic devices. He is unsure why they are doing this but believes that they wish to harm him in some way. He feels that he needs protection but is unsure who he can trust. Tetsuya denies any previous psychiatric history. Psychiatry team discussion with his local service and their records reveal he has had a previous admission on section 3 of the Mental Health Act (MHA), resulting in a diagnosis of schizophrenia. He was on a depot antipsychotic but appears to have disengaged from all follow-up 6 months ago He drinks 2 pints of lager on Friday, Saturday and Sunday evenings; no illicit substance use *MSE* **A**ppearance and behaviour: refusal to put down bag, muttering to himself **S**peech: normal **E**motion: alert, anxious **P**erception: possible hallucinations **T**hought content and process: paranoid ideation **I**nsight and judgement: none **C**ognition: distracted and unable to remember facts
Outcome	Tetsuya will need treatment for his psychotic illness and will require a MHA assessment
Reassess risks	He will need one-to-one observations in the department. Medications should be offered to help reduce his distress levels in the department. However, this may be refused. If he becomes more aroused and agitated, he will require review regarding potential need for restraint and rapid tranquillisation

Case 7.2				
45-year-old Naomi has been brought to the emergency department by her partner after increasing concerns regarding her strange behaviour over the last week. When she had returned from shopping, she found Naomi locked in the bathroom scared as 'some men had broken into the house and had been talking about hurting her'. There was no evidence of a break in. She was agitated and was holding a knife to protect herself. Her partner managed to remove the knife and ring for help.				
Primary assessment	ABCD	– Maintaining own airway – RR 24, saturations 100% in air – HR 120 irregular, BP 145/92 – Temperature: 37.8°C	AEIO	**A** – Agitated and anxious, pacing, paranoid **E** – In mental health room in ED **I** – No intent to harm self or others. Risk of absconding. Presence of irrational thoughts **O** – No objects now
SMART	SMART assessment – positive Suspected new-onset symptoms Abnormal vitals			
Unified assessment and immediate treatment	Medical assessment is required			
Secondary assessment				
Focused physical history and secondary examination	Increasing anxiety over the last week. Background history of weight loss and complaining about being too hot. No viral symptoms. Previously fit and well. On OCP ECG performed: atrial fibrillation. Bloods low normal, WCC raised, CRP normal. TFTs suggestive of hyperthyroidism (low TSH, High T3)			

Focused conversational psychological history and mental state examination (MSE)	No past psychiatric history of note No drugs of misuse, very occasional alcohol Reduced sleep recently with increasing anxiety. Had planned to see GP as this was upsetting her. Wondered if she was approaching menopause *MSE* **A**ppearance and behaviour: wearing tracksuit. Kempt. Restless and hypervigilant **S**peech: fast, difficult to interrupt **E**motion: anxious and suspicious, feels unsafe **P**erception: hears strangers in the house, probable auditory hallucinations **T**hought content and process: believes there are strangers in the house, held with delusional intensity **I**nsight and judgement: limited insight **C**ognition: orientated in time, person and place
Outcome	Seen side-by-side with emergency psychiatric team. Treated for thyrotoxicosis initially with beta-blocker. Diazepam for anxiety. Referred to medical team for further management
Reassess risk	Currently risks are medical and psychological because of delirium/psychosis secondary to thyrotoxicosis Risks communicated to medical team and nurses. While paranoid needs one-to-one care. Continued orientation and reassurance. Benzodiazepine PRN. Reassessment from mental health team. Continue management for thyrotoxicosis

7.11 Summary

As outlined in this chapter, it is important to ensure that organic causes are considered in the evaluation of an apparent mental health presentation. The SMART Form may be used to provide an approach to identify those patients who may need further medical evaluation.

The next two chapters cover two very important situations that have significant behavioral and physical health implications: alcohol and drugs of misuse and delirium.

CHAPTER 8

The apparently intoxicated patient

Learning outcomes

After reading this chapter, you will be able to:

- Identify how to rapidly and systematically assess the patient presenting with apparent intoxication
- Discuss diagnoses commonly mistaken for alcohol intoxication or alcohol withdrawal syndrome
- Describe risk factors for and management of alcohol-related brain injury
- Illustrate how illicit substance use can present as a psychiatric emergency

---

8.1 Introduction

Alcohol misuse is a major cause of morbidity and mortality in many countries and, as such, is ranked by the World Health Organization as one of the leading causes of burden of disease. Harmful use of alcohol is associated with 2.5 million deaths per year worldwide.

Europe is the heaviest drinking region in the world, with over 20% of the adult population reporting excess alcohol use. Over 20 million people are treated in Emergency Departments (EDs) in England each year, with a significant proportion of these visits being related to alcohol misuse at weekends. Over a million hospital admissions per year are associated with alcohol consumption, with a male : female ratio of 2:1. The cost to the UK National Health Service is estimated at £3.5 billion per year. It is well recognised that patients with severe mental health illness are more likely to misuse alcohol and drugs than the general population. A meta-analysis performed in 2022 showed that alcohol use is associated with a 94% increase in risk of death by suicide. It is therefore important that patients attending the ED with thoughts of suicide or

---

Acute Psychiatric Emergencies: A Practical Approach, Second Edition.
Edited by Mark Buchanan and Damien Longson.
© 2025 John Wiley & Sons Ltd. Published 2025 by John Wiley & Sons Ltd.

self-harm should be seen by the mental health team rather than the presentation being seen as 'just the alcohol'.

8.2 Alcohol by numbers: percentages, units and levels

Alcohol consumption is often recorded in units. A UK unit of alcohol is equivalent to 8 g/10 mL of ethanol. Cans, bottles and cartons of alcoholic drinks will often display alcohol content as a percentage. A bottle of whisky at 40% strength will contain 40 mL of ethanol per 100 mL The conversion process from percentage strength to units is outlined in the formula below.

Calculating alcohol consumption in units

$$\text{Units} = \text{percent alcohol}\,(\text{ABV}) \times \text{volume in mL}\,/1000$$

Worked example: a 750 mL bottle of wine at 12% strength: 12 × 750/1000 = 9 units

ABV, alcohol by volume.

8.3 The apparently intoxicated patient

Patients presenting with apparent alcohol intoxication can be a complex and challenging group in terms of assessment and treatment (Box 8.1). Acute disturbance is common, as are co-morbid injuries, attempted self-harm and medical conditions that require attention. It is not uncommon for diagnosis of intracranial bleeding to be delayed due to confusion being attributed to intoxication.

Box 8.1 Key priorities in the apparently intoxicated patient

- Rapid, systematic assessment for potentially life-threatening injuries and other physical health issues that require prompt treatment
- Consideration of thiamine replacement and treatment of substance withdrawal
- Identification and treatment of conditions that might mimic intoxication
- Screening for mental and physical health complications associated with chronic alcohol use
- Offering stabilised patients brief psychological interventions or signposting to suitable services where appropriate
- It is possible that first and foremost, de-escalation techniques and rapid tranquillisation may need to be deployed to enable assessment

8.4   Alcohol intoxication

Clues from the history

Consider how much time has elapsed since the patient originally presented (if several hours ago, their presentation should have improved at least in part). From the paramedic notes/collateral history gather as much information as possible.

- Where was the patient picked up?
- Was any alcohol found in their possession?
- Did they smell of alcohol?
- Was their presentation at that time suggestive of alcohol intoxication?
- Are there any presenting features on the paramedic history sheet that appear to have resolved or have things got worse (consider peak alcohol levels emerging, withdrawal or an evolving physical health problem)?
- Is there a history of previous presentations – if so what for?
- Is there a documented or collateral history of heavy alcohol use or illicit substances?
- Is there any psychiatric, medical or medication history that might provide clues to an alternative diagnosis or co-morbidities that should not be overlooked?

Features of alcohol intoxication overlap with some of the symptoms and signs suggestive of mental health problems such as mania and schizophrenia, but disturbed level of consciousness and cerebellar motor features are usually absent in the latter conditions. There are other conditions, however, that mimic the behavioural and motor features of alcohol intoxication, and these should not be missed. Intoxication with benzodiazepines or opioids can be mistaken for alcohol intoxication or they may have been co-ingested; it is important to try to confirm this as specific treatments exist that can rapidly reverse life-threatening features of intoxication. Other conditions that resemble alcohol intoxication are outlined later in this chapter.

Measuring drug/alcohol intoxication

The 2022 National Institute for Health and Care Excellence (NICE) guideline NG255 specifically states that you should not use breath or blood alcohol levels to delay psychosocial assessment. The guideline also states that if, when seen, it is felt that the patient is unable to partake in the assessment, they should have regular reviews by the mental health team to ensure this is done as soon as possible.

Studies have shown that most patients will self-report alcohol or drug use. Most patients, if asked in a sensitive way, will tell you what drugs they have recently taken. The reliability of patient self-reported drug use had a sensitivity of 92% and specificity of 91%. The reliability of self-reported alcohol use was 96% sensitive and 87% specific.

Urine drug testing has a significant false positive rate. The presence of drugs or alcohol in testing can lead to confirmation bias leading to important diagnoses being missed.

NICE describe alcohol dependence as 'a cluster of behavioural, cognitive and physiological factors that typically include a strong desire to drink alcohol, tolerance to its effects, and difficulties controlling its use. Someone who is alcohol-dependent may persist in drinking, despite harmful consequences, such as physical or mental health problems. If alcohol is stopped suddenly it can cause the patient to withdraw.'

8.5 Diagnoses commonly mistaken for alcohol intoxication (or alcohol withdrawal syndrome)

Intoxicated patients attending the ED is a common occurrence. However, there are many co-morbid presentations and conditions that mimic alcohol intoxication. It is important to consider common co-morbidities and alternative diagnoses (Box 8.2).

Box 8.2 Co-morbidities not to miss

- Head injury, including concussion
- Other traumatic injuries (falls, altercations, deliberate self-harm)
- Overdose
- Seizures
- Wernicke's encephalopathy
- Hallucinosis
- Suicidality
- Aspiration and respiratory tract infections
- Cardiomyopathy
- Gastritis
- Pancreatitis
- Hepatitis/cirrhosis
- Coagulopathy
- Ingestion of illicit drugs

Head injury deserves special consideration as it is a common co-morbid presentation and it is sometimes the correct underlying diagnosis in an apparently intoxicated patient. Important questions to ask include the timing and mechanism of injury, duration of any loss of consciousness, presence of seizures, vomiting, retrograde or anterograde amnesia and whether the patient takes anticoagulants. Examination should include Glasgow Coma Scale (GCS) score, cervical spine and neurological examination and inspection of face and scalp for signs of fractures.

In the UK, NICE has constructed guidelines to assist healthcare professionals making decisions in both pre-hospital and hospital settings about patients with suspected head injury. This includes guidance on whether a patient requires neuroimaging after head injury and how urgently this should take place (NICE guideline NG232, 2023).

8.6   Alcohol withdrawal syndrome

Alcohol withdrawal syndrome (AWS) and delirium tremens (DTs) can present with psychiatric symptoms. These can include anxiety, depression, suicidal thoughts and thoughts of self-harm. Patients can suffer from psychotic features such as hallucinations and delusions.

It is important to consider the risk of developing withdrawal symptoms while waiting as a result of delays associated with assessment or admission.

AWS can be defined as stopping or reducing alcohol (on the background of heavy prolonged drinking) associated with two or more of sweating, tachycardia, hand tremors, difficulty sleeping, nausea or vomiting, illusions or hallucinations that come and go, physical agitation, anxiety or seizures, where the symptoms are not attributed to another cause.

Those patients who are at risk of AWS include those who are drinking and have suffered from withdrawal previously, as well as those who suffer blackouts, have had seizures related to withdrawal or have suffered DTs in the past. It is important to remember that alcohol-dependent patients who are in hospital for a period of time may go through withdrawal as they no longer have access to alcohol.

8.7   Delirium tremens

Delirium tremens occurs in withdrawal from alcohol in patients who have been alcohol dependent for some time and is a medical emergency. It presents with clouding of consciousness including disorientation, recent memory impairment, tremulous hands, hyperhidrosis, severe agitation and insomnia. Patients describe or can be seen interacting with vivid and at times bizarre hallucinations. Often hallucinations are visual or somatic in nature; patients may report seeing or feeling spiders, snakes or even small figures (Lilliputian hallucinations). There may also be paranoid delusions. Physically, patients display autonomic dysfunction and dehydration with electrolyte disturbance, especially low potassium and magnesium levels. Symptoms, as with delirium, tend to worsen at night. DTs typically develops 24 hours after the last drink and lasts for up to 6 days.

The severity of alcohol withdrawal can be calculated by validated scores such as the Glasgow Modified Alcohol Withdrawal Scale (GMAWS) (Figure 8.1). There are other scores such as the Clinical Institute Withdrawal Assessment Alcohol Scale Revised (CIWA-AR).

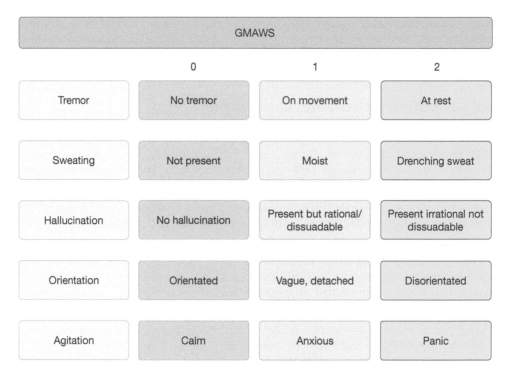

GMAWS			
	0	1	2
Tremor	No tremor	On movement	At rest
Sweating	Not present	Moist	Drenching sweat
Hallucination	No hallucination	Present but rational/ dissuadable	Present irrational not dissuadable
Orientation	Orientated	Vague, detached	Disorientated
Agitation	Calm	Anxious	Panic

Figure 8.1 GMAWS

The ongoing treatment of AWS sits outside the scope of this book, but the initial treatment is important. Benzodiazepines are the mainstay in management. Depending on the symptom severity and agitation of the patient, this can usually be managed with an oral benzodiazepine but in severe circumstances may require intramuscular or intravenous benzodiazepine therapy. Tranquillisation is sometimes required to keep the patient safe.

8.8   Alcohol-related brain injury

As well as AWS/DTs management, alcohol-related brain injury (ARBI) must be considered. ARBI encompasses Wernicke's encephalopathy and Korsakoff's syndrome.

Wernicke's encephalopathy is an acute neuropsychiatric disorder caused by thiamine deficiency. Thiamine is essential for cerebral metabolism and myelin sheath formation.

Patients with alcohol dependence often have a limited diet and alcohol directly reduces the absorption of what little thiamine they are ingesting. Alcohol dependence increases the risk of thiamine deficiency because of poor thiamine intake and absorption, poor thiamine storage and increased requirement. Thiamine is stored in the liver, which is impaired in alcohol-related liver disease. Finally, as well as reducing thiamine absorption, alcohol consumption increases demand for thiamine as it is used in its metabolism.

In the early stages of Wernicke's encephalopathy there is loss of appetite, nausea and vomiting, fatigue, diplopia, insomnia and anxiety and memory loss. Long-term signs and symptoms include oculomotor abnormalities, ataxia and confusion. The patient may be disorientated, with confabulation and hallucinations.

Patients with suspected Wernicke's encephalopathy should be given parenteral thiamine, and this should be seen as an emergency drug given early in the patient's care. The current best practice is that this should be given three times a day while in hospital. Oral thiamine should be considered if the patient is discharged. Ongoing management of Wernicke's encephalopathy is not in the scope of this course.

Wernicke's encephalopathy should be seen as a medical emergency as without treatment it has a mortality rate of approximately 15%, and 84% will go on to develop Korsakoff's psychosis.

Korsakoff's psychosis manifests predominantly as an inability to lay down new memories with coexisting retrograde amnesia. Patients confabulate (invent memories) for the episodes of amnesia. The patient is not trying to deceive or lie. They truly believe these memories. This is a devastating disorder leading to patients requiring long-term care.

8.9   Substances with potential for misuse

Drugs/substances of misuse

Often, intoxication with illicit substances leads to the development of psychiatric symptoms, particularly psychotic symptoms. Some of the more commonly encountered substances and effects are listed below.

Amphetamines (including methyl amphetamine) – may present as mania or psychosis. Psychotic symptoms often include delusions of insects being present under the skin with associated tactile hallucinations. Amphetamine-related psychosis can be expected to have significantly improved within a week of cessation of amphetamine use

Anabolic steroids – mood instability, aggression, depression and paranoia

Cannabis – both acute intoxication and chronic use may be associated with paranoia, psychotic symptoms and mood fluctuations

Cocaine/crack cocaine – initially euphoria followed by a period of dysphoria leading to hallucinosis and psychosis. Similar to amphetamine psychosis there may be delusions of insects under the skin and associated tactile hallucinations. The psychotic symptoms generally resolve within 24–48 hours

Diazepam – generally sedative effects but there may be paradoxical excitement and aggression

Ecstasy – generally feelings of euphoria, however psychotic symptoms have been reported with heavy use

Ketamine – derealisation and depersonalisation, paranoia and psychotic symptoms

Khat – elation and psychotic symptoms when heavily used

Lysergic acid diethylamide (LSD) – labile mood, synaesthesia, vivid hallucinations and illusions, which tend to be visual. Altered sense of time and space may be accompanied by distortions of body image. The effects are short lived lasting up to 16 hours, however LSD-induced psychosis may last several weeks and, in some reports, years

Magic mushrooms (psylocybin, psilocin) – predominantly hallucinations

Opiates, buprenorphine, methadone – sedative effects and depression. Psychotic symptoms have been reported with buprenorphine and methadone

Phenyclidine (PCP) – psychotic symptoms which can be associated with violent behaviour

Solvent abuse – euphoria, disinhibition and hallucinations

Novel psychoactive substances

Drugs generally act on specific receptors, particularly dopamine (the 'reward' system) and serotonin (involved in mood, anger and perception); other receptors including opioid and cannabinoid receptors may also be involved.

Novel psychoactive substances (NPS) are modern drugs (Figure 8.2), usually synthesised in a laboratory, and typically based on more traditional recreational drugs including heroin, cannabis, amphetamines and ketamine. However, a particular challenge relating to NPS is that one drug may cause multiple effects and can often act very differently at different doses.

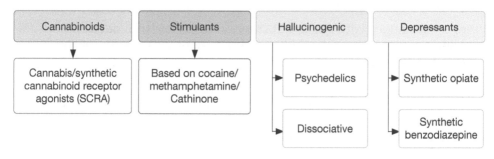

Figure 8.2 Novel psychoactive substances

Synthetic cannabinoid receptor antagonists (SCRA) are especially known for causing behavior-related attendances at EDs. Cannabis itself contains cannabidiol (CBD) and tetrahydrocannabinol (THC). THC is the more psychoactive substance of the two. CBD has anxiolytic and antipsychotic properties. Cannabinoids tend to only have THC and are purely psychoactive leading to psychosis, agitation and confusion.

Stimulants and hallucinogens can acutely cause psychotic episodes, agitation, and anxiety episodes.

8.10 Case example

Case 8.1

Karl is 42 years old. Police were called to an altercation outside a bar. On arrival, Karl is sitting against a wall, initially drowsy and confused, with a minor wound to his forehead and vomit next to him. Witnesses state he was involved in an argument and a short scuffle occurred. There is no history of loss of consciousness. He refuses to give details of his medical and mental health history. The police called an ambulance. When a paramedic attempted primary survey, Karl roused, became aggressive and refused to be assessed; he appeared sweaty and tremulous. The paramedic is querying intoxication. Whilst drowsy, the paramedic and triage nurse are able to perform limited assessment.

Primary assessment	ABCD	**A** – Maintaining own airway, RR 24, reluctant to be examined **B** – Oxygen saturations 98% on air, non-compliant with chest examination **C** – Clammy peripheries, HR 102 bpm, BP non-compliant, capillary refill 2 seconds **D** – GCS 12/15, dilated pupils, no obvious focal neurology, apyrexial, whilst drowsy rapid fingerprick performed: glucose 2.8 mmol/L	AEIO	**A** – Currently aggressive (verbally aggressive in ED and history of possible recent assaultative behaviour from police) **E** – In cubicle, ligature free, single door. Police have left **I** – When roused, expressing wish to leave **O** – Has a bag of possessions in the cubicle with him. Unsure whether this has been searched for objects that may be a risk
SMART		**S**MART assessment – positive **M**edical condition – diabetes **R**isky presentation – intoxication/head injury		
Unified assessment and immediate treatment		Physical health – GCS 12 (eyes: open to speech; verbal: confused, aggressive response; motor: will not obey commands) Once roused, aggressive demeanour. Capillary blood glucose level indicates hypoglycaemia. Patient has refused cannulation and oral Glucogel but is willing to drink sugary drinks. Head wound cleaned and dressed. CT head scan requested but non-compliant – consider capacity, observation level and contingency plan for treatment of acute agitation. Parallel assessment is required. Karl currently lacks capacity to make informed decisions on investigations and treatment		

Secondary assessment	
Focused physical history and secondary examination plus investigations	Compliance improves gradually after oral glucose and he allows bloods. Currently complains of mild headache and some dizziness. Accepts oral paracetamol. Karl confirms diagnosis of type 1 diabetes with frequent episodes of hypoglycaemia. Remainder of systems examination is unremarkable. Repeat blood glucose is just below normal range ECG – normal CT brain – delayed awaiting further assessment once glucose in normal range
Focused conversational psychosocial history and mental state examination (MSE)	GCS improves to 14/15 after glucose Karl has not tried to harm himself No history of cognitive impairment, major affective or psychotic disorder No recent life events Describes a longstanding history of hazardous drinking. Patient confirms he has not taken any illicit substances or overdosed on prescribed medications. Karl admits to getting into a fight with three men and has a history of convictions for assault when intoxicated *MSE* **A**ppearance and behaviour: now compliant and cooperative **S**peech: mildly slurred **E**motion: mood now normal **P**erception: normal **T**hought content and process: normal, admits has been drinking **I**nsight and judgement: has insight, accepts need for treatment and observation **C**ognition: some cognitive slowing in keeping with residual effect of intoxication
Outcome	Admit for overnight neurological observation. Glucose levels monitored, review by diabetes specialist nurse and alcohol/substance team
Reassess risks	No concerns about immediate risk to self Now more settled – risks to self and others low Engagement with care – currently willing to remain in hospital and receive investigations and treatment
Handover	Summarise presentation, key findings and current treatment plan using SBAR

8.11   Summary

It is important to consider alcohol and drugs of misuse as a cause of the psychiatric presentation. This can be due to acute intoxication or because of withdrawal. Joint assessment is still beneficial and is backed by both the *Side by Side* document and NICE self-harm guidance.

CHAPTER 9

The acutely confused patient

Learning outcomes

After reading this chapter, you will be able to:

- Recognise key features of the acutely confused patient
- Describe how to screen for delirium and consider alternatives
- Identify how to investigate reversible causes of delirium
- Demonstrate how to implement a comprehensive management plan

---

9.1 Introduction

Acute confusional states are a common emergency presentation in the Emergency Department (ED) or general hospital setting. Presentations can be diverse, as are the range of underlying causes. As discussed in Chapter 7, an important early distinction that should be made is whether confusion is part of a primary mental health presentation (such as mania or psychosis) or is associated with a potentially reversible cause (such as electrolyte imbalance or sepsis). There are many cases where the distinction is unclear (examples include acute-on-chronic confusional states, effects of illicit drug intoxication/ withdrawal and overdoses). The primary focus of this chapter is recognition and management of delirium. This includes assessment of alternative presentations such as affective and psychotic disorders.

Acute Psychiatric Emergencies: A Practical Approach, Second Edition.
Edited by Mark Buchanan and Damien Longson.

9.2 Acute confusional states

Delirium

Delirium is a complex, organically driven neuropsychiatric presentation characterised by disturbance of multiple cerebral functions. These include level of arousal, attention, perception, motor behaviour (e.g. agitation, retardation, tremor, asterixis, myoclonus), sleep–wake cycle, emotion and cognitive functions such as memory, language and visuospatial abilities.

Specific patient populations have been highlighted as being particularly susceptible to delirium (Table 9.1). Most studies report data from later life patients (>65 years) but delirium can occur across age groups and may be a pointer of physiological disturbance.

Table 9.1 Pooled point prevalence of delirium in different patient populations in the general hospital setting

Population	Frequency
Postoperative	35–65%
Oncology	25–47%
General medicine	10–35%
Acute respiratory failure	37%
Stroke units	2–66%
Intensive care unit – on admission	7–30%
Intensive care unit – during admission	60–80%
Patients with dementia	18%
Presentations to ED	8–17%
Admissions from ED	14–24%

Impact of delirium: the case for early recognition and treatment

Delirium has been shown to adversely affect prognosis, hence timely diagnosis and early treatment are essential. Four mechanisms have been suggested that link delirium to long-term neural impairment:

- Direct neuronal damage as a consequence of delirium
- Indirect effects of altered neurotransmitter concentrations and receptor sensitivity
- Acceleration or diversion from normal neurophysiological ageing
- Exacerbation of pre-existing impairments

Delirium is associated with an increased risk of secondary infections, falls, prolonged hospital stays, loss of independence (increased rates of discharge to more supportive settings), long-term cognitive impairment and a threefold increase in 6-month mortality rates. Delays in diagnosis and treatment of delirium in the intensive care unit (ICU) are associated with increased mortality in this patient group.

- Delirium is **common** among acutely unwell patients
- It has **serious** immediate *and* long-term implications
- It remains **underdiagnosed** and **undertreated**

Recognising delirium: key features

A multicentre survey of UK junior doctors highlighted that although most were aware of the high prevalence and potential seriousness of delirium, many found diagnosis and acute management challenging.

Although you are less likely to meet them in an acute mental health emergency, do not dismiss the patient who is described as 'pleasantly confused'. Delirium can present as hypo- or hyperactivity and both represent an acutely unwell patient with a high risk of increased morbidity and mortality.

Specific diagnostic criteria can be found in the American Psychiatric Association's *Diagnostic and Statistical Manual of Mental Disorders*, 5th edition (APA, 2013) and the World Health Organization's *International Classification of Diseases*, 11th edition (WHO, 2022).

Important things not to miss in the assessment

Is there any suspicion here of self-harm? If so, proceed to the SLIPA risk assessment. If there is no suspicion of self-harm, proceed to the remainder of the focused psychosocial history.

Undertake a clinical assessment for delirium:

- History from staff, relatives and notes to set the presentation in context
- Key symptoms
- Confusion developed over hours, days, weeks or months?
- Different to baseline?
- Fluctuates during the course of the day?
- Disturbed sleep–wake cycle?
- History of cognitive impairment – diagnosis?
- History of mental health problems?
- Alcohol excess – any sweating/tremor over the last few days?
- Illicit drug misuse?

The checklist in Box 9.1 is a distillation of both sets of diagnostic criteria.

Box 9.1 Delirium diagnostic checklist

1. The current presentation should be different to the patient's baseline, have developed over hours to days (occasionally weeks) and should fluctuate in severity during the course of a day
2. There should be clouding of consciousness – reduced clarity of awareness of environment ('spaced out', drowsy)
3. Attention is disturbed (directing, focusing, sustaining and shifts of attention). Answers to questions might be frankly irrelevant or more subtle impairments where patients focus initially but quickly become distractible or perseverative. Impaired attention and concentration may prevent adequate assessment of other cognitive functions
4. There may be additional disturbance of one or more cognitive domains – immediate recall and recent memory and disorientation in time and place are most commonly affected. Other cognitive domains that may be affected include language (appropriate understanding and production), visuospatial ability (e.g. planning and drawing a clock), perception (misinterpretations and hallucinations) or a combination of these. Bedside cognitive tests commonly used include the AMT (abbreviated mental test) and the MoCA (Montreal cognitive assessment), which includes a version for visually impaired patients
5. There may be psychomotor disturbance (rapid, unpredictable shifts from hypo- to hyperactivity; may also manifest as sustained periods of hyper- or hypoactivity)
6. There may be disturbance of the sleep–wake cycle (insomnia, daytime somnolence, reversal of sleep–wake cycle, nocturnal worsening of symptoms, disturbing dreams that may continue as hallucinations or illusions after waking)
7. Symptoms should not be better explained by the presence of other pre-existing or evolving neurocognitive disorders such as learning difficulties or dementia
8. There might be evidence that physiological disturbance from a general medical condition, intoxicating substance, toxin, medication or a combination of these are directly responsible for the confusional state. An important caveat is that the cause may not be found in up to 15% of patients

Supportive features
- Emotional disturbances (depression, anxiety, fear, irritability, euphoria, apathy or perplexity) are common but not specific for diagnosis
- Transient delusions (often persecutory in nature) are sometimes present

Screening tools

There are many rapid screening tools for delirium.

The 4AT (Figure 9.1) is a brief and effective screen that focuses on alertness, orientation, attention and fluctuations. It is highly sensitive and specific. It is proven in routine care, with high completion rates and delirium detection at expected clinical rates.

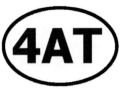

(label)

Patient name:

Date of birth:

Patient number:

_____

**Assessment test
for delirium &
cognitive impairment**

Date: Time:

Tester:

CIRCLE

[1] ALERTNESS
*This includes patients who may be markedly drowsy (eg. difficult to rouse and/or obviously sleepy
during assessment) or agitated/hyperactive. Observe the patient. If asleep, attempt to wake with
speech or gentle touch on shoulder. Ask the patient to state their name and address to assist rating.*

Normal (fully alert, but not agitated, throughout assessment)	0
Mild sleepiness for <10 seconds after waking, then normal	0
Clearly abnormal	4

[2] AMT4
Age, date of birth, place (name of the hospital or building), current year.

No mistakes	0
1 mistake	1
2 or more mistakes/untestable	2

[3] ATTENTION
*Ask the patient: "Please tell me the months of the year in backwards order, starting at December."
To assist initial understanding one prompt of "what is the month before December?" is permitted.*

Months of the year backwards

Achieves 7 months or more correctly	0
Starts but scores <7 months / refuses to start	1
Untestable (cannot start because unwell, drowsy, inattentive)	2

[4] ACUTE CHANGE OR FLUCTUATING COURSE
*Evidence of significant change or fluctuation in: alertness, cognition, other mental function
(eg. paranoia, hallucinations) arising over the last 2 weeks and still evident in last 24hrs*

No	0
Yes	4

4 or above: possible delirium +/- cognitive impairment
1-3: possible cognitive impairment
0: delirium or severe cognitive impairment unlikely (but
delirium still possible if [4] information incomplete)

4AT SCORE [   ]

GUIDANCE NOTES   Version 1.2. Information and download: **www.the4AT.com**
The 4AT is a screening instrument designed for rapid initial assessment of delirium and cognitive impairment. A score of 4 or more
suggests delirium but is not diagnostic: more detailed assessment of mental status may be required to reach a diagnosis. A score of 1-3
suggests cognitive impairment and more detailed cognitive testing and informant history-taking are required. A score of 0 does not
definitively exclude delirium or cognitive impairment: more detailed testing may be required depending on the clinical context. Items 1-3
are rated *solely on observation of the patient at the time of assessment*. Item 4 requires information from one or more source(s), eg. your
own knowledge of the patient, other staff who know the patient (eg. ward nurses), GP letter, case notes, carers. The tester should take
account of communication difficulties (hearing impairment, dysphasia, lack of common language) when carrying out the test and
interpreting the score.
Alertness: Altered level of alertness is very likely to be delirium in general hospital settings. If the patient shows significant altered
alertness during the bedside assessment, score 4 for this item. **AMT4 (Abbreviated Mental Test - 4):** This score can be extracted from
items in the AMT10 if the latter is done immediately before. **Acute Change or Fluctuating Course:** Fluctuation can occur without delirium
in some cases of dementia, but marked fluctuation usually indicates delirium. To help elicit any hallucinations and/or paranoid thoughts
ask the patient questions such as, "Are you concerned about anything going on here?"; "Do you feel frightened by anything or anyone?";
"Have you been seeing or hearing anything unusual?"

Figure 9.1 4AT: assessment test for delirium and cognitive impairment form
Source: 4AT – Rapid Clinical Test for Delirium (the4at.com)

Another commonly used tool worldwide is the confusion assessment method (CAM). Box 9.2 shows the CAM criteria for delirium. Pooled sensitivity and specificity are generally encouraging (82% and 99%, respectively). Sensitivities are variable across different patient populations however and, as such, a focused clinical assessment remains the gold standard.

Box 9.2 CAM criteria for delirium

- Confusion that has developed suddenly and fluctuates, *and*
- Inattention — ask if the person is easily distracted or has difficulty in focusing attention, *and either*
- Disorganised thinking — ask if the person's thinking is disorganised, incoherent, illogical or unpredictable (e.g. they have an unclear flow of ideas, change subject unpredictably or have rambling or irrelevant conversation), *or*
- Altered level of consciousness — ask about changes in level of consciousness from alertness to lethargy (drowsy, easily aroused), stupor (difficult to arouse), comatose (unable to be aroused) or hypervigilant (hyperalert)

Primary psychiatric disorders as a cause for confusion

Patients with psychiatric conditions such as bipolar affective disorder or schizophrenia can appear acutely confused during relapse, although consciousness is not usually impaired and fluctuations are perhaps less acute. Generally speaking it is very unusual for primary psychiatric presentations to change within hours or days. Changes in a mental health condition usually change over weeks and months. A sudden change from baseline should be suspected to have a physical health aetiology in the first instance. Whilst it is possible, developing a new schizhophrenia or other psychotic condition in later life is considerably less common than a delirium.

Conversely, psychotic symptoms (i.e. where somebody has lost contact with reality through either hallucinations or delusional beliefs) are very common in delirium. The nature of the psychosis is often paranoid and very distressing. Patients commonly have visual hallucinations and delusional beliefs.

Depressive pseudodementia

If a confused patient appears hypoactive, enquire about symptoms of depression, especially depressed mood, feeling unable to enjoy anything, feeling guilty or worthless and thoughts of life being pointless. Note that in depressive pseudodementia, attention and concentration are usually normal but the patient may require prompting to continue with a task as they may give up early. As discussed earlier, if it is a sudden change then consider a hypoactive delirium.

Acute exacerbations of chronic condition

Patients with chronic cognitive impairment (developmental disabilities or neurodegenerative disease such as dementia) can also present with acute confusion and behavioural change. This may be related to disease progression – patients with vascular dementia can experience sudden deterioration in cognitive function post-infarct (note this may represent delirium *or* disease progression) – or disease fluctuations – dementia with Lewy bodies follows a naturally fluctuating course.

Social and environmental stressors such as alterations or more restrictive routines can cause agitation, distress and acute behavioural change. It is also important to consider whether the presentation you see in front of you is an expression of fear or distress. Think about whether there may be safeguarding issues.

Key points

For patients with chronic cognitive impairment:
- Acute cognitive and behavioural change may represent natural fluctuations or disease progression but exclude delirium FIRST
- This is a vulnerable patient group. Be alert to the possibility of safeguarding issues

---

Precipitants of acute confusion

Working out the precipitants of acute confusional states can be tricky as often there are multiple contributing factors. The principal aim of the emergency assessment is to screen for potentially life-threatening reversible causes in addition to gaining an impression of risk of harm to the patient and to others. It is also helpful to think of predisposing risk factors that render a patient susceptible to developing acute confusion (Table 9.2) and what perpetuating factors might hinder recovery (Table 9.3).

Table 9.2 Causes of delirium		
Precipitating factors I: general causes	**Precipitating factors II: intoxication, toxicity, withdrawal and deficiency states**	**Precipitating factors III: primary neurological disease**
Trauma	Alcohol, sedatives	Head injury
Hypoxia/hypercapnia	Illicit substances	Bleed (subdural haematoma, subarachnoid haemorrhage)
Ischaemia	Delirogenic drugs	
Infection	Polypharmacy	Stroke
Electrolyte disturbance	Overdose	Non-convulsive status epilepticus or post-ictal state
Hyponatraemia	Exposure to toxic substances	
Hypercalcaemia	Renal failure	Meningitis
Hypermagnesaemia	Liver disease (hepatic encephalopathy, hepatitis, liver failure)	Viral or autoimmune encephalitis
pH disturbance (lactate, ketones, etc.)		Vasculitis (e.g. systemic lupus erythematosus)
	Malabsorption and/or malnutrition: vitamin B_1 or B_{12} deficiency	
Uraemia		Primary or secondary malignancy
Hypoglycaemia		Raised intracranial pressure
Thyroid or adrenal disease		
Constipation and/or urinary retention		

Table 9.3 Factors that increase the risk of delirium and hinder recovery	
Predisposing factors	**Perpetuating factors**
Advanced age	Pain
Vascular risk factors	Dehydration
Cardiac disease	Constipation
Pulmonary disease	Sensory impairment
Cognitive impairment	Insomnia
Sensory impairment	No clock or visible daylight
Co-morbidity load	No visits
History of alcohol or illicit drug misuse	Noisy, stimulus-rich ward
	Low staff : patient ratio

9.3 Preparation

Establish key concerns at this moment – does current risk exist?

Acute confusion and current risk

The patient has acute cognitive and behavioural change coupled with:

- Agitation and distress
- Aggression including attempts to harm self or others
- Wandering and falls
- Bags packed and trying to leave the hospital
- Refusing oral intake
- Refusing essential medical/nursing input such as observations, investigations and/or treatment

The focus here is diagnosis and acute management of risks.

Reason for presentation to ED

Gather any collateral information from paramedics, police or accompanying others (where was the patient found, who called the ambulance, duration of confusion?):

- Acute departure from patient's usual baseline
- Any physical health symptoms or signs
- Initial Glasgow Coma Scale (GCS) score
- Physical observations
- Any associated features including aggression or refusal to come into hospital

There should be a brief review of the latest observations and medication chart (blood tests and electrocardiogram (ECG) if readily available).

> **Key point: medication review**
>
> Beware drugs with sedative properties (antihistaminergic, GABAergic, opioids), high anticholinergic load or those with toxicity syndromes. Common culprits include tricyclic antidepressants, bladder stabilisers, digoxin, carbamazepine, antiparkinsonian medications, opiates and non-selective β-blockers.

Box 9.3 has guidance on engaging the acutely confused patient.

Box 9.3 Engaging the acutely confused patient

- Think about sensory impairments and language barriers
- Introduce yourself and explain why you are here, using clear, simple language
- Express concern and reassure you are here to help
- Adopt a friendly, polite, concerned approach
- Try to make eye contact (shift position if necessary to make this easier) but do not stare – this can be intimidating
- A light touch on the arm or shoulder can help a confused patient to focus and engage but can also irritate or startle a suspicious or agitated patient – use your judgement and consider your personal safety
- Deal with risks first but spending a few seconds acknowledging the patient's fear/irritation/upset can open a window of communication and ultimately negotiation regarding further assessment, taking bloods, etc.
- When a patient wanders from topic, use the patient's first name, re-establish eye contact and use a polite segue back to your question/topic, for example *'Jack, I just want to ask about . . ./Can you tell me if you are . . .'*

Legal capacity

Does the patient have the capacity to consent to examination, investigation and the management plan? Do they have the capacity to decide to remain or leave? Do they have capacity to make an informed decision on this? Should they be assessed anyway in their best interest?

Psychotic experiences

Psychotic experiences are common in delirium.

Does the patient appear to be responding to non-apparent stimuli (looking at, gesturing towards or talking to unseen people/creatures/objects)? Do they appear unduly agitated, suspicious or frightened? Do you have any concerns that the risks identified previously or a desire to leave the department are driven by psychotic symptoms such as command hallucinations or paranoid delusional beliefs?

Next steps

This will be based on specific identified risks (to self, others or risk of leaving the department). The mainstay of treatment at this stage is: (i) providing support and monitoring from members of nursing staff; (ii) sedative medication as and when required if unduly agitated and distressed; and (iii) highlighting psychosis to the ED team as it may inform further investigation in patients without an established prior history of psychosis.

9.4   Emergency management: principles of shared care

Teams should share the following perspectives if they have assessed in parallel:

- **Physical health team:** Is there any evidence of a physical health problem or toxic/withdrawal state that could explain the current presentation? If so, what is the working diagnosis and plan for further investigations and treatment?
- **Mental health team:** Is delirium the most likely explanation for the confusional presentation? Are there any psychiatric co-morbidities to consider? Are substance misuse or alcohol dependency contributing to/ likely to impact on this presentation? What risks to self and others have been identified? What is the immediate plan for managing these?
- **Both teams:** Has the patient's capacity to consent to or refuse to remain in hospital to have further investigations and treatment been established? If an extremely agitated, unwell patient is refusing further input and lacks capacity, an urgent joint plan must be implemented that enables action in the patient's best interests. This commonly involves rapid tranquillisation to reduce distress and agitation and to enable further investigation and treatment. On rare occasions, colleagues from intensive care may get involved as intubation and ventilation may be required to administer life-saving treatment.

9.5   Determine outcome

1. **Delirium most likely and examination and investigations point to a probable cause:** Admit to a general hospital setting for further investigation and treatment. Ongoing input from liaison psychiatry is needed to review progress, and to advise on managing risks and discharge planning.
2. **Delirium most likely cause and examination and investigations are normal:** Admit to a general hospital setting to commence further investigations. Ongoing input from liaison psychiatry is needed in terms of suggesting/further discussion of relevant investigations, management and review of progress.
3. **Delirium unlikely and examination and investigations are normal:** Seek a psychiatric opinion regarding possible transfer to a mental health setting or discharge with intensive support if risks are low and the patient assents to further assessment and treatment.

9.6   Ongoing care plan

The following pharmacological and non-pharmacological strategies may be helpful when formulating care plans.

Non-pharmacological measures

Nurse in a moderately lit room if possible and try to provide a day/night light cycle. A night light can be helpful as it allows sleep but helps the patient reorient more quickly if they do not wake to complete darkness. Try to avoid room changes.

Depending on the level of agitation and distress and associated risks to self and others, one-to-one support may be required. The member of staff doing this should take a proactive approach to reorientate the patient several times a day (day, month and year, time, location, reason for being in hospital, name of key member of staff), engage in conversation, reassure, monitor input and output and check the patient is comfortable. Daily brief screens can also be carried out such as the CAM or 4AT.

Calendars, signs and clocks can help orientation. Correct sensory impairment where possible (glasses, dentures and hearing aids are often mislaid).

Early mobilisation has also been shown to hasten recovery from delirium. Non-ambulatory patients should be referred to physiotherapy for help with maintaining muscle and joint integrity.

Monitor hydration and pain levels. Check for and tackle urinary retention and constipation.

Involve relatives and carers and explain what is going on. It is important to mention that delirium can take time to resolve – often days to weeks but occasionally months.

Pharmacological measures

For persistent, severe agitation and/or distress associated with hallucinations and delusions try on an as required basis first. If beneficial, consider writing up regular doses once or twice daily but ensure this is reviewed frequently. Drugs to consider are haloperidol, olanzapine, risperidone and quetiapine.

Try to avoid benzodiazepines unless delirium was precipitated by drug or alcohol withdrawal. Chlordiazepoxide, oxazepam and diazepam are typically used in these patients. If it becomes necessary in other patient groups (concerns arise about using antipsychotics, etc. or they are not available in an urgent situation) use a short-acting version such as lorazepam.

9.7   Handover

Risks should be reassessed, and essential information regarding presentation, working diagnosis and treatment plan should be collated for handover to the receiving team.

9.8 Case example

Case 9.1				
A 66-year-old woman, Lyla, has been brought into the ED by paramedics. It is winter and her neighbour saw her in a summer dress in her garden. On approaching her, she appeared confused and distressed, asking where her husband is. The neighbour was under the impression that she was divorced and lives alone. Whilst compliant with paramedic assessment, she refuses cannulation and oxygen. She is a heavy smoker and has a history of type 2 diabetes, chronic kidney disease stage 3 and previous myocardial infarction. There is a previous history of depression.				
Primary assessment	ABCD	**A** – Maintaining own airway **B** – RR 29, oxygen saturations 88% room air (normal saturation levels unknown), crepitations right lower and middle lung zones **C** – HR 105 bpm, normotensive **D** – Pyrexial 38°C, fingerprick glucose 9 mmol/L	AEIO	**A** – Confused. No concerns currently regarding active plans to self-harm or harm others **E** – Wandering around department **I** – No obvious intent to harm self or others, moderate risk of leaving due to confusion, some evidence of irrational thought **O** – No dangerous objects
SMART	**SMAR**T assessment – positive **S**uspected new onset **M**edical conditions – diabetes, kidney disease, heavy smoker **A**bnormal vitals **R**isky presentation – age over 55			
Unified assessment and immediate treatment	Physical health – clinical evidence and notes indicate probable respiratory infection (sepsis). Investigations and treatment performed under the Mental Capacity Act and best interest. Contingency plan for treatment of acute agitation Working diagnosis: delirium secondary to respiratory tract infection			
Secondary assessment				
Focused physical history and secondary examination plus investigations	In hospital records, her next of kin is not her husband but her son, who lives in Australia. She continues to be confused and difficult to manage. Contact number for son rings out but it is night time in Australia. She becomes distressed and angry when nurses attempt to persuade her to comply with investigations/treatment			

Focused conversational psychosocial history and mental state examination (MSE)	*MSE* **A**ppearance and behavior: now in hospital gown, history of inappropriate clothing **S**peech: normal, mainly quiet **E**motion: emotionally labile **P**erception: normal **T**hought content and process: disordered **I**nsight and judgement: no insight regarding need for treatment and remaining in hospital **C**ognition: impaired
Outcome	Any ongoing further treatment must be done with a consideration of the Mental Capacity Act and best interest Fortunately, son answers his phone. Speaks to mother once a week and last contact was 6 days ago. At that call, states she had complained of a history of lethargy, increasing shortness of breath, right-sided pleuritic chest pain and cough with green sputum. Had seen GP and just been commenced on treatment Son agrees to FaceTime with mum in department. As a result, she becomes more trusting of the medical staff and clinical management CXR – right side consolidation lower and mid zones Admit to general hospital under care of physicians with mental health liaison team support, if required
Reassess risks	Risks as in primary assessment (unchanged)
Handover	Summarise presentation, key findings and current treatment plan using SBAR

9.9 Summary

Acute confusion is common and may represent a warning flag for an acute medical or mental health emergency. It is important to exclude delirium first and foremost. A collaborative approach between ED/ward staff and the mental health liaison team is essential for rapid identification and effective management.

CHAPTER 10

The aggressive patient

Learning outcomes

After reading this chapter, you will be able to:

- Characterise the risk factors for aggression in hospital settings
- Demonstrate how to assess for aggression/violence
- Identify how to manage aggression/violence
- Identify the early signs of the patient who is becoming angry or violent
- Describe how to approach and communicate with the patient
- Recognise how to de-escalate a potential aggressive situation

---

10.1 Introduction

Circumstances leading to violence and aggression can occur in clinical settings for a variety of reasons. Workers in healthcare and social assistance experience higher rates of non-fatal assaults than workers in other industries. Assaults most commonly occur in the Emergency Department (ED) and psychiatric units. Surveys undertaken by ED nurses have reported up to 100% experiencing verbal assault and over 80% physical assault in their previous year at work (May & Grubbs, 2002).

It is therefore essential that practitioners know how to recognise early signs of violence, are able to assess these situations at the earliest opportunity and de-escalate any aggression that occurs. There should be subsequent opportunity for debrief, support and reflection, for patients and staff.

It is important that early signs of behavioural or emotional change are taken seriously, sensitive attention drawn to these changes, and appropriate support and actions taken. While staff in psychiatric hospitals have provision for

---

Acute Psychiatric Emergencies: A Practical Approach, Second Edition.
Edited by Mark Buchanan and Damien Longson.
© 2025 John Wiley & Sons Ltd. Published 2025 by John Wiley & Sons Ltd.

training in understanding changes in others – allowing them to pre-empt aggression – staff working within general hospital settings may lack this guidance. Without this expertise, situations may escalate rapidly, or a staff member may become unknowingly drawn into a potentially violent situation. Professionals with experience and background in the recognition and prevention of aggression should therefore be proactive in assisting and training those without.

10.2   Principles in assessing aggression and violence

The Royal College of Psychiatrists has outlined recommendations for assessing and managing risk to others (RCPsych, 2017), with essential points included here (Box 10.1).

Box 10.1 Recommendations about assessing harm to others

- Risk cannot be eliminated, but it can be rigorously assessed and managed or mitigated
- It is important to identify a history of violence or risk to others
- A risk assessment should pinpoint key factors that identify risk is increasing
- Risk is dynamic, it can be affected by circumstances that change over the briefest of timeframes. Risk assessment needs to include a short-term perspective and frequent review
- Some risks are specific, with identified potential victims
- Specialist risk assessment may be required (e.g. sex offending)
- Risks to children must be explicitly considered
- Effective communication is a key part of any risk management plan
- Clear communication of the risk assessment outcome and management plan is essential
- Patients who present a risk to others may also be vulnerable to other forms of risk (e.g. self-harm, self-neglect, retaliation or exploitation by others)

   In addition, transparency in reporting incidents and the duty of candour should always be considered.

What is aggression?

Aggression refers to harmful physical or verbal behaviour (or threats) towards persons or objects. Violence refers to the resultant action. Professionals working in ED and psychiatric settings may be frequently called to assess, evaluate and manage aggression (either as a main concern, or secondary to the presenting complaint). However, it should never be thought of as relating only to patients. Aggression can originate from any person, including staff, visitors or other professionals. The causes of aggression presenting in an emergency setting are often multifactorial and complex – resulting from biological, social, cultural and medical factors. Although there is a perception that mental illness is associated with aggression, the link between psychiatric illness and aggression is contentious and disputed. Furthermore, the perception that poor mental health is automatically associated with violence can reinforce stigma for vulnerable distressed patients, leading to exclusion or lack of appropriate care.

Theories of aggression

The determinates and causes of aggression and violence are not well understood. However, an understanding of the main theories of aggression can be used to help predict situations where aggression may occur, enabling management and a plan for prevention.

Possible causes of aggression

The causes of aggression related to psychiatric disorders (from studies by Foley, 2005 and Bjørkly, 1995) are outlined in Box 10.2.

Box 10.2 Causes of aggression related to psychiatric disorders

- Co-morbid substance misuse
- Non-adherence to medication
- History of childhood abuse
- Involuntary admission status
- Lack of insight
- Previous history of violence
- Younger age
- Male sex
- Organic brain disorders
- Learning disability

Association between aggression and mental illness

Violence as a result of mental illness remains rare. Currently, it is understood that severe psychopathology can be a cause of aggression and violence, with risk deemed highest the closer the proximity is to the first psychotic episode – especially if this is associated with delusions. This is an important consideration when assessing a person with a newly suggested diagnosis of psychosis. However, the MacArthur Violence Risk Assessment Study (MVRAS) (Monahan, 2008) indicates that delusions do not predict violence. It needs to be stressed that patients who are mentally ill are more likely to be victims of violence than perpetrators; they experience violence outcomes at higher rates than the general population.

Use of substances and their relationship with aggression and violence

Substance misuse has been shown to be a risk factor for aggression and violence (Soyka, 2000). Substance misuse can increase the risk of psychotic symptoms and medication non-adherence, which in turn may lead to worsening of symptoms, greater impulsivity and a corresponding increased risk of violence (Pickard & Fazel, 2013). Intoxication with alcohol can also increase the risk of violence and aggression.

Location, environment and the risk of aggression

Environments that are busy, disorganised and chaotic elevate stress levels for all involved, increasing the risk of misunderstanding and aggression. Any patient being admitted to a hospital who finds themselves disorientated, without privacy and unable to leave, is at a potentially higher risk of becoming frustrated and angry. If there are significant delays in finding a mental health bed, this directly increases the risk of agitation. Additionally, if a patient has attended for a specific purpose and these concerns are not listened to and addressed this can lead to frustration leading to aggression.

Staff variables associated with aggression and violence

Poor communication (or lack of communication) is a central component when aggressive incidents escalate (Yap et al., 2023). Hospitals have placed emphasis on improving communication, but the increased pressure on staff and resources means there may be limits and constraints to providing communication that is timely and effective. Negative staff attitudes to certain patients can also result in stigma, a perceived lack of care and resultant aggression.

Communication skills are an important aspect of the structured approach. Good communication between doctor and patient can reduce psychological anxiety. Good communication can 'improve a patient's perception of the medical encounter regardless of treatment outcome' (Pfeiffer et al., 1998). However, poor communication can 'thwart the goal of understanding patient expectations of treatment or involving the patient in treatment planning' (Baile et al., 2000).

10.3   Risk formulation

The Royal College of Psychiatrists' report *Assessment and Management of Risk to Others* (RCPsych, 2017) outlines that 'risk formulation' encapsulates an understanding of personality, mental state, environment, potential causes, protective factors and any corresponding changes to these. Aim to answer the following questions:

- How serious is the risk?
- How immediate is the risk?

- Is the risk specific or general?
- How volatile is the risk?
- What are the signs of increasing risk?
- Which specific treatment and/or management plan can reduce the risk?

Risk and confidentiality

When assessing risk, consent to risk assessment should be sought and an explanation of the risks and benefits of the process given. Patients should be made aware of confidentiality and the situations when information may be shared without their consent.

The General Medical Council (GMC, 2018) outlines five situations when information can be disclosed:

- The patient consents, whether implicitly or explicitly for the sake of their own care or for local clinical audit, or explicitly for other purposes
- The patient has given their explicit consent to disclosure for other purposes
- The disclosure is of overall benefit to a patient who lacks the capacity to consent
- The disclosure is required by law, or the disclosure is permitted or has been approved under a statutory process that sets aside the common law duty of confidentiality
- The disclosure can be justified in the public interest

The Royal College of Psychiatrists' report *Assessment and Management of Risk to Others* (RCPsych, 2017) also gives guidance regarding sharing patient information. Patient-identifying information may be shared:

- With the patient's explicit consent
- On a need to know basis when the recipient needs the information because they will be involved with the patient's care (where staff from more than one agency are involved, the patient needs to be told that some sharing of information is likely)
- If the need to protect the public outweighs the duty of confidentiality to the patient

10.4   Managing potential aggression and violence

The risk of aggression and violence should be considered in the assessment of any patient. All professionals have a responsibility to take adequate steps to reduce risks and remain aware of signs of aggression or frustration.

Hospital, patient and staff variables can all contribute to aggression. Each of these will be addressed in turn. It must be stressed that in numerous studies no clear definitive indicator has been proven to predict specific risk and therefore a global approach aiming to reduce risk across multiple domains is advocated.

Hospital variables

It is essential that the environment for the patient assessment is appropriate.

Steps to reduce risk include:

- All interview rooms should have a panic alarm system and multiple doors allowing access and exits
- Items that could be used as potential weapons should not be available
- Steps should be taken to ensure that patients are not interviewed on isolated corridors or in ill-lit areas
- The interviewer must always alert another professional to their whereabouts and a system must be in place to ensure that someone can be contacted immediately
- If a patient is intoxicated or under the influence of substances, steps should be taken to allow both the patient and attending staff to be kept safe until a time when an interview is possible
- The patient should be asked about possessing weapons or substances on their person

Steps to improve engagement and rapport should also be taken:

- The patient should be interviewed in an appropriate setting with adequate privacy
- The patient should be orientated as to where they are, why they are there and who they are talking to. The patient should also be aware of who to contact to obtain further information
- The patient should not be made to feel overwhelmed or trapped
- Provision should be made for breaks, food and drinks
- Waiting times should be addressed. If there is a delay, then clear communication of the expected wait must be made

Patient variables

Certain characteristics amongst patients and their experiences indicate a higher likelihood of violence and aggression. If possible, these should be identified and assessed, prior to interview, from records, collateral history and other professional sources. If a collateral history cannot be obtained, these variables should be explored tactfully during the consultation.

- Assessment should include a patient's narrative of their own risk. The patient's agenda and needs are listened to and as far as possible addressed
- Gender: men are more likely than women to commit violence with a higher possibility of this resulting in the victim requiring medical treatment and the arrest of the perpetrator
- Age: young patients are more likely to be aggressive. However, a subgroup of elderly patients with organic disorders (dementia, delirium) are also at higher risk of committing physical violence to others
- Previous violence: previous violence can be a predictor of future violence; therefore the patient's forensic history should be checked prior to assessment with collateral information obtained if possible
- Childhood experiences: negative experiences as a child (childhood maltreatment, physical, sexual abuse or neglect) may be linked to violent

relationship in adults (Jennings et al., 2011) and increased risk of substance misuse (Gutierres & Van Puymbroeck, 2006). Furthermore, a parental figure who misused substances or has a forensic history increases the risk of a child perpetrating violence in the future

- Diagnosis: a substance misuse diagnosis is strongly indicative of a risk of aggression and violence
- Psychopathy: a diagnosis of antisocial personality disorder is strongly indicative of a risk of violence
- Delusions: the presence of delusions alone are not predictive of violence. However, if the content of these delusions are persecutory, the risk of aggression increases
- Hallucinations: specific command hallucinations instructing a violent act are associated with an increased risk of violence
- Thoughts: ruminating on persistent violent thoughts increases the risk of aggression
- Anger: the more anger displayed by the patient, the higher the risk of violence towards others

Staff variables

- Staff must be alert to the early risk signs of aggression
- Staff should be appropriately trained in de-escalation
- Staff who are rigid and authoritarian in their manner are at increased risk of violence. Furthermore, staff who expect violence are found to be at higher risk
- Junior staff must have the support of seniors, and should not be left to deal with escalating situations alone (care assistants and student nurses are found to be those most assaulted in studies)
- Reduced staff turnover improves the relationship between staff and patients
- Handover and meal times are noted to have higher levels of violent incidents
- A protocol should be available outlining how to deal with the aggressive client, with a code of conduct and consequences for violence

10.5 Assessment, prevention and management of risk

Assessment

A risk assessment should be carried out including a review of the patient's history, forensic history, the characteristics of the current admission and the current mental state of the patient. McAllister and Patel (2012) define risk assessment as 'the systematic collection of information from all sources to estimate the degree to which harm (to self or others) is likely at some point in time'. It is a dynamic process and can change at any time.

Within the structured approach (see Chapter 1), risk should be a consideration at all stages, with risk assessment a key component of the **U**nified risk assessment and handover segments.

As outlined in Chapter 2, the person who is acutely disturbed should have a primary assessment that is designed to identify and manage any immediate risk to safety. This involves a risk assessment alongside (where appropriate) a rapid assessment of airway, breathing, circulation, disability (neurological status). A full discussion of this approach is covered in Chapter 2.

Prevention

Preventing the escalation of risk can be divided into three stages: primary prevention, secondary prevention and tertiary prevention (Figure 10.1).

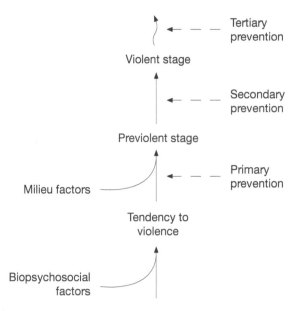

Figure 10.1 Assessment and prevention

Primary prevention

This involves identifying and controlling (as far as possible) hospital variables, patient variables and staff variables outlined earlier in this chapter.

Secondary prevention

This involves employing measures at the 'pre-violent stage'. At this stage aggression is increasing and the patient is at higher risk of violence. Variables outlined in primary prevention may no longer be able to be addressed; the focus switches to an immediate reduction in risk.

Early recognition of this stage and prompt de-escalation are essential.

Agitation can escalate at any time due to changes in patient, staff and environmental factors. Therefore, the variables outlined in Section 10.4 should be reviewed and reflected on, even when a situation has been de-escalated.

The most effective use of de-escalation is the completion of pre-emptive steps prior to and during the interview so that agitation is minimised. The skilled practitioner will be aware of factors that may contribute to escalation, with the emphasis on risk reduction.

If agitation does increase despite initial attempts at reducing risk, then the principle of a non-coercive approach should be at the forefront of any actions taken.

The competent practitioner will be ready to step back and consider an alternative approach (Box 10.3). This can be done either during the interview or by having a physical 'time out' for all parties.

- The practitioner should attempt to identify if any part of their interview style is contributing to the escalation. Medical interviews can sometimes take on a paternal or domineering tone. If recognised, this can be addressed by asking the patient again for their views or goals, directing the interview back to a collaborative approach.
- Goals for all parties should be regularly addressed throughout the interview. A patient may become agitated if they feel they are not receiving an outcome or being listened to. Equally, the interviewer may become terse or display less empathy if they are worried about time pressure or the call of their bleep. A relative may feel they are being prevented from either returning home or going to work.
- Instead of viewing a patient as 'difficult' or 'uncooperative', staff should employ empathy, recognising and acknowledging the reasons for a patient's frustration. The interviewer should also self-reflect; they may be doing as well as possible under the circumstances or their behaviour may be a reinforced response to previous difficult ED encounters. If recognised, this will reduce the chances of this situation playing out in the same negative way as those past interviews.
- Patients should be offered alternatives to aggression or violence allowing them to 'save face'. If a patient's normal reaction to stress is aggression, it should be positively acknowledged when they are not displaying aggression in a stressful situation. Respect should be shown for remaining non-violent, enabling positive reinforcement of alternative behaviours and reducing the perceived threat of lost dignity (Gertz, 1980).

When using verbal de-escalation, it is better to approach it as a loop rather than a straight line. It may be necessary to return to basic principles at many points during the interview, for example checking the patient is aware of exactly who you are and why you are present. This re-establishes goals and assists orientation (important if the patient has been waiting for several hours).

> ## Box 10.3 Alternative approaches to environment and interaction
>
> - Review if the room is well lit, quiet, offers a calm environment and is not isolated. If the room is not suitable and is adding to patient or staff frustration, address this openly. It may not be possible to find alternative clinical space, but having this conversation with the patient can demonstrate mutual understanding of the challenges of the situation
> - Intense triggers should be removed or reduced (this may include other people)
> - Are the chairs and environment detrimental to the situation? Does the patient feel they are trapped, overly scrutinised or surrounded? Are chairs and staff situated behind the patient so the patient cannot see all participants? Is the patient at a lower level (on the floor/on a mattress) while staff are standing? Attempt to address issues such as these
> - Body language and posture are important. Do not stand over the patient or adopt an aggressive stance. Maintain a neutral facial expression, mirror the patient's posture and maintain intermittent (non-staring) eye contact. Reflect if your tone is overly authoritative, strict or critical (possibly reminding the patient of childhood experiences)
> - Have you offered information to both the patient and relatives? Has this been understood? Does this need to be offered again (hint: it is advisable to stop and summarise every 10–15 minutes to allow all present to understand what is happening, for patients and staff)

Aim for an interview and communication approach that is engaging, non-judgemental and collaborative (Box 10.4).

Certain skills are used in successful de-escalation situations: staff are perceived to be open, honest, supportive, self-aware and non-judgemental. They can maintain self-control even in situations of high anxiety (allowing the patient to feel secure), and they are aware of verbal and non-verbal cues (Price and Baker, 2012).

Richmond et al. (2012) outline reasons why verbal de-escalation should be considered prior to the use of medication or physical restraint:

- If staff members use physical restraint it may reinforce to both the patient and staff that force or violence is a necessary step to resolve agitation
- Patients physically restrained are more likely to be admitted to a psychiatric ward and have, on average, longer periods of in-patient stay
- If verbal de-escalation is used then patients and staff are less likely to be harmed

Box 10.4 Verbal approach to de-escalation

- Introduce yourself clearly, explaining why you are present. Ask the patient why they are there and their aims and intentions. Outline your own objectives, emphasise the positive but do not hide potential difficulties
- Help the patient to orientate to the situation. Clocks, newspapers and media can be used to aid this process
- Use common words, short sentences and display a calm manner
- Establish limits, for example the possible duration of the interview
- Set limits of acceptable behaviour and explain these 'ground rules' in advance. Explain that violence is not acceptable
- Use active listening, summarise and reflect back what the patient is saying
- Involve the patient in a collaborative dialogue with shared problem solving
- Encourage the expression of feelings and emotions
- Discourage acting out and importantly do not be drawn into punitive reactions
- When communicating a decision explain clearly and simply with space for reflection and questions. Be optimistic and provide hope
- Return to patient and staff goals and check if they have been addressed

Tertiary prevention

Tertiary approaches involve management of violence.

If the patient remains aggressive despite attempts at communicative and environmental de-escalation, then alternative approaches may be necessary. It is important to continue to consider the 'loop' principle of de-escalation (outlined earlier): can parties pause and return to primary and secondary approaches?

If a patient is violent, consider what steps need to be taken to support the patient rather than excluding them from care. Exclusion can leave the patient (or other members of the public/professionals) at increased risk.

Physical intervention

An unwell patient may require the presence of security to protect themselves and others. Any manual restraint should be undertaken by staff who work together closely as a team with an understanding of roles and a clearly defined team lead:

- Manual restraint should never be used that interferes with a patient's airway, breathing or circulation
- Alternatives to manual restraint should be considered, for example pharmacological medication
- An ED is not a mental health ward and therefore close working with trained mental health staff is essential. Ongoing safety reviews concerning the best location to manage and support the patient should be undertaken

A physically and mentally well member of the public who becomes violent or agitated can be excluded from the ED and the police contacted. It is important to consider the longitudinal impact of this on the person, staff and other members of the public.

Pharmacological intervention

- Medication can be offered in an oral form to an agitated patient to help calm anxiety and prevent the need for physical intervention:
  - A small dose of a benzodiazepine can be offered orally
- If oral medication is refused and the use of intramuscular medication required, the following need to be taken into account:
  - Coexisting physical issues
  - Patient's advance wishes and directives
  - Current prescribed/non prescribed use of medications or substances
  - Previous reaction to medication and allergies

Rapid tranquillisation is covered in Section 10.7.

After use of a restrictive intervention, a post-incident debrief should be conducted and this should involve multidisciplinary staff, including security if they were involved.

- Factors leading to the incident should be investigated
- The current status of the incident should be addressed
- Plans should be made to reduce the chance of a similar incident occurring in the future and strategies to reduce this incident of aggression formulated
- The patient should be given an opportunity to discuss the incident
- Necessary documentation should be completed in a timely manner

10.6   Case examples

Case 10.1

A 29-year-old man, Kieran, presents to the ED. He is demanding that he is given a prescription of methadone. He informs reception that he received his usual dose of 40 mg methadone yesterday, but the chemist is shut today and he lost his prescription. Reception tells him he will have to wait to be seen at which point he becomes quite abusive, telling her he feels like he is going to die and can't stop sweating and shaking.

Primary assessment	ABCD	**A** – Maintaining own airway **B** – RR 22, oxygen saturations 95% **C** – HR 105 bpm, BP 130/89 **D** – No neurological deficit, pupils moderately dilated, apyrexial	AEIO	**A** – Becoming agitated when he has to wait **E** – In the ED waiting room **I** – Not expressing intent to self-harm. Threatening to leave if he is not seen quickly **O** – Has not been searched
SMART		**SMAR**T assessment – positive **S**uspected – withdrawal from opioids **A**bnormal – tachycardia, moderately dilated pupils **R**isky presentation – withdrawal symptoms and potential escalation of aggression		
Unified assessment and immediate treatment		Physical health – judged to be at the early stage of withdrawal, however can wait for assessment by a clinician Mental health – angry, not an immediate risk of physical violence to self or others, but risk of escalation. Ongoing risk of verbal aggression. Risk of absconding. Needs to be asked regarding potential objects on person This patient requires de-escalation of anger and aggression, with clear communication of a plan for medication		
Secondary assessment				
Focused physical history and secondary examination		Known drug dependence on methadone support. Physically the patient is presenting with early signs of drug withdrawal consistent with a missed dose of methadone. Demanding immediate dose of opiate to overcome withdrawal Plan to confirm previous dose and dispensing history with named pharmacy and to re-establish current regime. In the meantime he can be given symptomatic medication		

Focused conversational psychosocial history and mental state examination (MSE)	Known to community drug services and confirmed as being on a methadone support programme after years of intravenous heroin use. Presents as angry and demanding without thought for others *MSE* **A**ppearance and behavior: sweating and shaking, agitated, aggressive **S**peech: raised volume, mild pressure, able to interrupt **E**motion: mild lability and emotional change **P**erception: nil elicited **T**hought content and process: logical form and content **I**nsight and judgement: reasonable insight **C**ognition: orientated to time, place and person, has capacity regarding request for medications
Outcome	Arrange immediate support for his drug withdrawal with a plan for ongoing community biopsychosocial support for his dependency
Reassess risks	With plan for medication review in place, risk to self and others is reduced Engagement with care – currently willing to remain in hospital and receive medication outcome Minor risk of absconding if time delayed, therefore regular communication with patient and review of any agitation essential
Handover	Summarise presentation, key findings and current treatment plan using SBAR

Case 10.2

Gemma, a 26-year-old woman, is brought to the ED by her husband. She had given birth to a boy 7 days ago via a difficult, painful, forceps delivery. She is currently presenting in the department as highly agitated and dressed in mismatched clothing. When approached by staff (especially females) she is abusive and not making any sense. Her husband states he is now exhausted trying to look after his wife and child. Gemma states she must leave the department to carry out the aliens' work which involves her newborn son.

Primary assessment	ABCD	**A** – Maintaining own airway **B** – RR 20, oxygen saturations 96% **C** – HR 98 bpm, BP 120/80 **D** – No neurological deficit, PERLA, apyrexial	AEIO	**A** – Agitated, irritable with delusional thoughts. Risk to others including her own infant **E** – In mental health room **I** – Wishes to leave but not actively attempting to do so **O** – No dangerous objects
SMART		**SM**ART assessment – positive **S**uspected – new-onset postpartum (puerperal) psychosis **M**edical conditions – early postnatal period (need to exclude infection/delirium) **R**isky presentation – risk of neglect of self and infant		
Unified assessment and immediate treatment		Physical health – infection and other physical complications need to be excluded Mental health – mental health emergency; consider capacity/detention to secure maternal psychiatric unit; urgent medication review; security required to prevent leaving and self-neglect Sensitive attention to an agitated patient, who is also a new mother, her bond with baby and potential need for safeguarding ED and psychiatric staff managing a mental health emergency (postpartum psychosis) supporting a very unwell mother and consideration of safeguarding issues for child		
Secondary assessment				
Focused physical history and secondary examination		Physical health – assessed by on-call medic and no acute concerns identified on examination. Blood tests, urinalysis and swabs later returned as within normal limits ECG undertaken in view of need of psychotropic medication – normal sinus rhythm		

Focused conversational psychosocial history and mental state examination (MSE)	Confirmed deterioration of mental health since birth with associated insomnia. Significant decline in the past 24 hours with severe lability of mood, confusion and agitation *MSE* **A**ppearance and behavior: wearing mismatched clothing, looks exhausted, agitated, asking to leave, possibly visibly responding **S**peech: spontaneous, raised volume **E**motion: confused, labile affect **P**erception: none admitted but visibly responding to possible auditory hallucinations **T**hought content and process: delusions about aliens **I**nsight and judgement: lacks insight **C**ognition and capacity: does not have capacity to make decision to leave or care for child
Outcome	The patient requires immediate treatment for a severe mental illness One-to-one security should be requested Medication (antipsychotic and benzodiazepine) sought for distress and acute treatment, under guidance from perinatal psychiatry as well as discussions with her mental health midwife and health visitor Assessment undertaken to ascertain the need for detention under an appropriate mental health provision Consideration should be made for admission to a maternal psychiatric unit Collaborative discussion (involving patient if possible, and family if consented) regarding safeguarding and professionals' meeting arranged
Reassess risks	The overall risk profile in this case is high for both patient and child Patient has a postpartum psychosis which involves delusional beliefs about her child There is a high risk of harm to either the patient or child via direct or indirect means
Handover	Summarise presentation, key findings and current treatment plan using SBAR

10.7 Rapid tranquillisation

What is rapid tranquillisation and when should it be used?

Rapid tranquillisation refers to the use of medication in patients presenting with agitated, disturbed and potentially dangerous behaviour, in order to calm the patient and prevent injury to themselves or others. Rapid tranquillisation is used when both psychological techniques and environmental management have failed to be effective. It is important to note that while the term rapid tranquillisation conjures up a picture of restrained patients being given intramuscular injections, where possible all medication should be offered orally first and given with the patient's consent.

The guide here applies to adult patients. There are certain patient groups where particular care must be taken. These include elderly, frail patients, those patients with coexisting physical illness, those who are intoxicated, pregnant women and those with learning disability. Physical illnesses that are most relevant include: head injuries, hypoglycaemia, drug overdose or respiratory failure (where tolerance may be reduced and signs of toxicity missed) and liver failure (where metabolism is reduced). In all such cases there are many variables that would alter the choice and dose of medication as well as the post tranquillisation monitoring regime.

Before prescribing medication for rapid tranquillisation you should consider where the patient will be placed for monitoring of both mental and physical health as well as the frequency of this monitoring. You should ensure that there are adequate resuscitation facilities. As most of the drugs that are used are short acting you will need to plan how the patient will be managed in the longer term. This may include prescribing regular medication and moving the patient to a more appropriate setting. It is also wise to plan for the possibility that the patient may require restraint or further sedation, and to make sure that staff are available should this be required.

It is vital at all times that the patient's dignity is respected. Even if the patient appears not to be able to understand information, an explanation of what is happening should be given throughout. Afterwards, when the patient is calm, it is often helpful for a member of staff to talk through what has happened with the patient.

As far as possible consider the patient's wishes when prescribing. If there is an advance directive or clear preference for a particular medication expressed by the patient, then use this if it is safe to do so and appropriate to the situation. Rapid tranquillisation can be given when justified using the legal frameworks surrounding capacity, common law and the power to provide medical treatment in particular circumstances. It is not possible in this book to outline individual jurisdictions' legal capacity arrangements, however it is worth pointing out that health professionals should assess and record a patient's capacity (on an ongoing basis) and indicate how they are acting in the patient's best interests if the patient is not deemed to have capacity.

Note if the patient is likely to require further regular medication (e.g. antipsychotics) to manage their psychiatric condition, and if they are not consenting to this then they will need assessment and detention under legal powers (e.g. the Mental Health Act if working in England) before this can be administered. On the other hand, when patients retain capacity and are not legally detained, then rapid tranquillisation may be appropriate but can only be given with their consent.

Prescribing for rapid tranquillisation

The aim of rapid tranquillisation is not to anaesthetise the patient but to mildly sedate ('tranquillise') them to a state where they are calmer, more reasonable and less distressed.

If a patient initially refuses oral medication and requires IM medication it is always worth taking both the injection and the tablets to the patient. Many, when faced with the choice that one or the other is going to be given, will agree to take the medication orally. Please note this process should not be a threatening one, the aim is to act in a patient's best interests and show them the options available, with the aim of them making the choice. The focus remains on a discussion between oral and IM medication.

If an injection is required, always ensure the injection site is exposed rather than injecting through clothing – there have been many occasions where the restraining staff have been accidentally injected rather than the patient.

Furthermore, situations can commonly arise with the following complications. Awareness and instruction in local protocol is essential.

- There is limited information about the patient
- The patient is antipsychotic naïve
- The patient suffers from cardiovascular disease and/or prolonged QT
- No electrocardiogram (ECG) has been completed

The need for investigations should be balanced against the immediate risk to patient and others, requiring clinical judgement. It is not in the scope of this book to outline specific medications or regimes as these will differ by area, trust and policy.

Your local policies and standard operating procedures will indicate preferred medications (and the concurrent investigations and physical reviews required).

Medication regimes

Titrate doses where possible (initial doses for the elderly may need to be substantially lower).

- Use specific drugs to treat target symptoms
- If polypharmacy is used, consider the rationale for this, the potential interactions and increased side effects
- Use the safest routes of administration
- Implement a regular treatment regime following rapid tranquillisation to enable ongoing reduction in symptoms and distress

Adverse effects and monitoring

Following the administration of IM medication all patients should be monitored regularly until such time that the level of consciousness is stable, blood pressure, respiratory rate and pulse are normal, and the patient is not complaining of any severe adverse effects such as dizziness on standing or dystonia.

The following should be monitored:

- Pulse
- Blood pressure
- Respiratory rate
- Temperature
- Level of hydration
- Level of consciousness

Monitoring should occur at least every hour until there are no further concerns about the service user's physical health status (follow local protocol).

Check the above every 15 minutes (more frequently, if deemed necessary) if the British National Formulary maximum dose has been exceeded or if the patient appears to be asleep or sedated, has taken illicit drugs or alcohol, has a pre-existing physical health problem, has experienced any harm as a result of a restrictive intervention, or is high risk, such as in pregnancy or elderly patients.

Undertake appropriate investigations (e.g. blood tests, ECG). There will, of course, be occasions where it is impossible to obtain an ECG or blood investigations, or the patient has physical risk factors. In these situations, you will need to balance the risks of tranquillisation with the risk of a patient continuing to suffer a disturbed and agitated state. This may prevent appropriate treatment for the underlying cause or lead the patient to act violently and recklessly. Junior doctors should obtain senior advice. Ensure that you document fully the reasons for your decision either to administer or not to administer medication and ensure that an appropriate monitoring plan is in place and that resuscitation equipment is available.

Pregnancy

See Chapter 11.

Common drugs used in intravenous tranquillisation

A wide range of drugs are available for rapid tranquillisation, depending on local protocol, practice and custom. These include haloperidol, olanzapine, risperidone, aripiprazole, lorazepam, promethazine, ketamine and droperidol. There is further information in an excellent systematic review by Castro et al. (2024).

Refer to your local hospital policy or national guidance.

Summary of rapid tranquillisation

Following psychological de-escalation and engagement techniques it may be necessary to prescribe medication intended to rapidly produce a state of tranquility and mild sedation. This reduces the risk of inadvertent harm, violence or inability to cooperate with vital assessment and treatment. As far as possible this should be with the consent of the patient and be explained and negotiated with appropriate choices given.

Figure 10.2 shows an example of an algorithm for rapid tranquillisation. It is important to use your own Trust's guidelines.

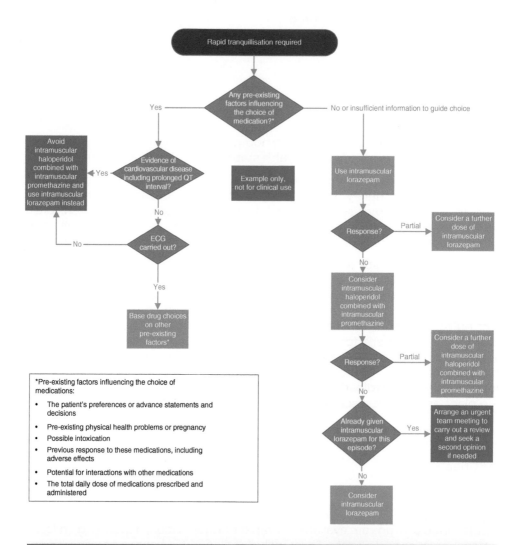

Figure 10.2 An example of a rapid tranquillisation flowchart. Please note this algorithm is for illustration purposes only and should not be used. Refer to local standard operating procedures for your drugs and doses

10.8 Summary

Aggression and violence can occur in any hospital situation, from a variety of sources (patient, professional, staff or family). Therefore, all staff working in a hospital should have an awareness of this risk. Aggression and violence are more common in ED and psychiatric settings than other parts of the hospital.

Each hospital should have a protocol to allow staff to assess aggression and violence in a structured clinical non-judgemental approach. Note, even a high-quality assessment may be ineffective unless there are clear instructions for immediate action and longitudinal management, and this is clearly communicated with all involved.

Risk cannot be completely eliminated, and this is not a desirable aim of any protocol as it may lead to inflexible and defensive practice. Responsible clinical risk taking (weighing up potential benefits and harms) should be encouraged.

Primary intervention should focus on precipitating background, staff and environmental factors to identify variables that may contribute to violence. Measures should be taken *in advance* to reduce and mitigate these variables.

Secondary intervention focuses on de-escalating an aggressive situation via communication skills (verbal and non-verbal). Effective communication is an essential aspect of de-escalation; education and training on communication skills should be prioritised.

Tertiary intervention focuses on the management of the aggressive patient, including physical and pharmacological means. This should also incorporate a reflection and debriefing stage for both patient and staff.

CHAPTER 11

Special considerations

Learning outcomes

After reading this chapter, you will be able to:

- Discuss considerations for children and young people, long bed waits and the Emergency Department, perinatal mental health, eating disorders and Safety Planning

---

11.1 Children and young people

The initial assessment of the patient with a mental health emergency mental health crisis is principally the same. The Unified approach (ABCD/AEIO) is still appropriate. It will identify the medical emergency and the psychiatric risks to the patient and others that may require intervention.

In the psychosocial assessment of the young person, HEADSSS (Figure 11.1) is a useful tool to identify risks that may be affecting the safety and mental health of the child. In all parts of the conversation, it is important to think about the young person's safety and to consider safeguarding issues throughout. The mental health of the patient may not warrant emergency intervention, but the social aspects may negate actions to keep the patient safe.

As ever this is not a tick box exercise but a framework to support a conversation.

It is always important to consider non-psychiatric causes for behavioural presentations. This is more so if the child is under the age of 12 years or the symptoms are of sudden onset. Other flags should include visual or tactile hallucinations, seizures and the absence of a family history of mental illness.

Acute Psychiatric Emergencies: A Practical Approach, Second Edition.
Edited by Mark Buchanan and Damien Longson.
© 2025 John Wiley & Sons Ltd. Published 2025 by John Wiley & Sons Ltd.

Example of things to address

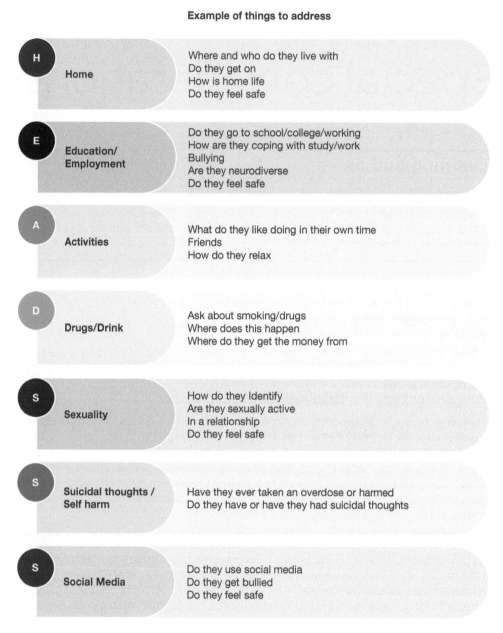

H	**Home**	Where and who do they live with Do they get on How is home life Do they feel safe
E	**Education/ Employment**	Do they go to school/college/working How are they coping with study/work Bullying Are they neurodiverse Do they feel safe
A	**Activities**	What do they like doing in their own time Friends How do they relax
D	**Drugs/Drink**	Ask about smoking/drugs Where does this happen Where do they get the money from
S	**Sexuality**	How do they Identify Are they sexually active In a relationship Do they feel safe
S	**Suicidal thoughts / Self harm**	Have they ever taken an overdose or harmed Do they have or have they had suicidal thoughts
S	**Social Media**	Do they use social media Do they get bullied Do they feel safe

Figure 11.1 HEADSSS

11.2   Long bed waits and the Emergency Department

Patients who are awaiting a mental health bed in the Emergency Department (ED) or on a medical ward are at risk of harm. Long waits increase the chance of patients absconding as well as aggression, agitation and violence.

In Acute Trusts, wards and the ED are not psychologically therapeutic environments. It is essential that the shared mental health and acute care continues.

The AEIO risk assessment is a dynamic one. Risk can change with time, as can the medical situation. It is imperative that patients have regular reviews both by the medical/emergency team and psychiatry.

The situation of patients waiting for a mental health admission may change. Admission may no longer be the least restrictive option or required. Conversely the patient may require a higher-level care bed such as in the psychiatric intensive care unit.

It is suggested that on each review by the psychiatric team the following is addressed:

- Level of supervision
- Current length of stay
- Legal status for hold – risk if the patient leaves
- Usual psychiatric medications
- Review the need for rescue interventions/medications (de-escalation/ restraint)
- Consideration of change to regular medications to reduce risk of need for de-escalation
- Recommendations
- Any other considerations

From a medical point of view, it is important to ensure that normal medications are prescribed including the consideration of venous thrombus prophylaxis. Any changes to the medical state of the patient should be addressed, for example the development of alcohol withdrawal.

11.3 Perinatal mental health

This is the time period from pregnancy to 1 year post delivery.

The Confidential Enquiry into Maternal Deaths (MBRRACE, 2023) showed that suicide is the leading cause of death in women from 6 weeks to 1 year post delivery. The method of suicide is usually by violent means such as hanging or jumping from a height. The enquiry also found that children are often not a protective factor, and this can be a false reassurance for professionals.

There are three red flags (Figure 11.2) which can help highlight women at risk.

Red flags

1. A significant change in mental state or emergence of new symptoms. These can occur very rapidly, sometimes within a day.

2. New thoughts or acts of violent self-harm

3. New and persistent expressions of incompetency as a mother, or estrangement from the infant

Figure 11.2 Red flags

There are also three amber flags (Figure 11.3) which make someone more susceptible to mental health problems and the associated risks.

Amber flags

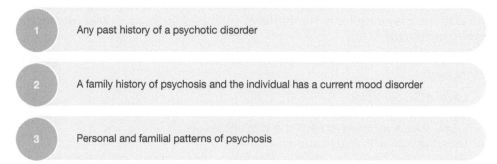

1 Any past history of a psychotic disorder

2 A family history of psychosis and the individual has a current mood disorder

3 Personal and familial patterns of psychosis

Figure 11.3 Amber flags

Self-harm in pregnancy or the early postpartum period is an unusual event, and should always prompt referral for continuing evaluation, ideally to specialist perinatal mental health services. If there are any concerns about someone who is in the perinatal period then seek a psychiatric review.

Accessing a perinatal bed

Across the country there are specialist mother and baby units. These are designed for women within the perinatal period who need an in-patient admission for their mental health. To help with ongoing bonding and attachment to their infant, the mother is admitted with her baby. To avoid delays in admissions, and to prevent separation of mother and infant, access to perinatal beds is national.

De-escalation in pregnancy

During pregnancy you need to consider carefully both risks to the mother and baby. If restraint or seclusion is required, the standard procedures will need to be modified to avoid harm to the mother and baby. Perinatal advice should be immediately sought with close collaboration between ED, the obstetric team, perinatal psychiatry team and, in later pregnancy, the neonatology team. When choosing medications, drugs with a short half-life are preferable. The minimum effective dose should be used. The choice of medication should be made with the advice of a perinatal psychiatry professional. Consideration should be given to potential effects of medication at different stages of the pregnancy and at delivery, for both baby (e.g. neonatal withdrawal) and mother (e.g. sedation). Any changes to medication or maternal care should also instigate a review and appropriate changes to the maternal birth plan (in collaboration with the patient).

When rapid tranquillisation is used, the relevant obstetric, neonatal and perinatal teams should be involved to assess what maternal/fetal /newborn monitoring is required.

11.4   Eating disorders

There has been an increase in presentations of patients (adult and children) presenting with the complications of eating disorders. The patient may present and share information that they or their friends or family are concerned about their eating. The symptoms can include change in weight and self-induced vomiting (either physically self-induced or by misusing laxatives and diuretics).

The Royal College of Psychiatrists has produced the *Medical Emergencies in Eating Disorders: Guidance and Recognition and Management* (MEED) guidelines (RCPysch, 2022) which made recommendations to improve the management of patients presenting with eating disorders.

Physical risk assessment should include nutritional status (including current intake), disordered eating behaviours, physical examination, blood tests and electrocardiography.

Patients who require admission to medical or paediatric wards should be treated by a team with experience of treating eating disorders. Plans should involve their carers. The MEED guidelines recommend that management protocols should be developed in collaboration with eating disorder specialists. Staff should be trained to implement them.

The medical team looking after the patient should manage refeeding safely. Rapid refeeding can cause refeeding syndrome; conversely underfeeding syndrome can be caused by too cautious refeeding. Purging behaviours can lead to fluid and electrolyte imbalance, these should be managed safely. The team should also work closely with psychiatric experts to decide on further management.

Mental health teams should support the medical teams dealing with the behavioural challenges common in patients with eating disorders. They should also be leading the discussion as to whether there is a need to assess and treat patients under compulsion using relevant mental health legislation.

Successful support for an in-patient with an eating disorder requires close attention to the behavioural manifestations of the illness. These include:

- Avoiding weight restoration by drinking water, secret or micro-exercise, purging and other behaviours
- Self-harm and suicidal thoughts
- Co-morbid psychiatric conditions
- Aggression or other disturbed behaviour

Management of these behaviours may require additional measures, such as one-to-one observation, structured collaboration between staff and the patient using a care plan, regular multidisciplinary staff meetings and involving patients and carers.

The question is when this becomes a risk to life?

The MEED guidelines include a check list for clinicians to identify the need for an admission. This looks at the history, examination and investigation. Box 11.1 provides a summary of the checklist.

Box 11.1 Check list for red flags indicating severity of presentation

History
- Rapid weight loss >1 kg per week for two consecutive weeks in an undernourished patient
- Frequent vomiting
- Muscle weakness
- Little urine output
- Intractable constipation
- Suicidal thoughts

Examination
- BMI <13, or m%BMI <70 in patients <18 years
- Pulse <40°C
- Postural hypotension + recurrent syncope
- Core temp <35.5°C
- Muscle weakness (SUSS, HGS)*

Results
- Any significant ECG abnormality
- Hypokalaemia <2.5 mmol/L
- Hypoglycaemia glucose <3 mmol/L
- HbA1C >10%
- Hyponatraemia
- Urine specific gravity <1.010
- Low phosphate
- Raised transaminases

* Sit up, squat, stand (SUSS) test: the patient is asked to sit up from lying supine on a flat surface without using the hands, if possible.
Squat: the patient is asked to squat and to rise without using the hands, if possible.
BMI, body mass index; ECG, electrocardiogram; HGS, hand grip strength; m%BMI, mean percentage BMI.

Anyone with one or more red flags or several amber flags (see MEED guidelines) should be considered high risk and there should be a low threshold for admission.

High-risk refeeding management involves a diet of less than 20 kcal/kg/day. This is built up over days. It is important to monitor electrolytes twice daily. In the absence of high-risk factors the patient can be started on 50 kcal/kg/day. The aim is to increase weight by 0.5–1 kg a day.

The involvement of psychiatry in the ongoing management of the patient is essential. There can be behaviours increasing the risk to the patient; these include falsifying weight, disposing/hiding food and exercising. There can be thoughts of self-harm and suicide. This is not only a stressful time for the patient, but also the patient's family and loved ones. It is essential to deal with these stresses and anxieties. There is a need to assess and treat patients under compulsion using relevant mental health legislation (RCPysch, 2022).

11.5   Safety Planning

In many situations covered in the APEx course there is a need for joint assessment. There will be areas where the ongoing management will be best dealt with either by mental health or physical health colleagues. This does not mean that the other team will not be required further down the pathway.

If a patient is in the ED for any length of time it is important to continue to co-manage the patient. A Safety Plan is a list of positive actions that people, and others, can do to help the patient to navigate their suicidal thoughts more safely.

Safety Planning has been in routine use in several countries for well over 10 years. The use of Safety Planning now has general support in England and is included in the latest National Institute for Health and Care Excellence (NICE) guidelines for self-harm and is recommended by the Royal College of Psychiatrists. There is a growing body of international evidence based on multiple studies including a systematic review, meta-analysis and a large-scale cohort comparison study, which demonstrate the feasibility, safety and efficacy of Safety Planning.

The Safety Plan can be thought of as the mental health equivalent of putting on a car seatbelt. At times of distress or crisis it can be difficult to think clearly, so the idea behind Safety Planning is to prepare for the difficult times before they happen.

Personalised, specific and detailed Safety Plans have better outcomes. A person's Safety Plan should be like a fingerprint – totally unique to them. A Safety Plan is so much more than a piece of paper or an app. It can act as an invisible thread back to better times, when a person felt calmer and less distressed. It can reconnect a person to realistic hope to help them see the light at the end of the tunnel and that things can get better.

Because an overwhelmed brain needs simple and easily accessible information, a Safety Plan has a clear, stepwise structure. It is designed to help someone safely navigate intense feelings and can help interrupt suicidal thoughts or plans and stop things spiraling out of control. A Safety Plan has several sections and uses a person's strengths and assets. It starts with the most helpful, easy or quick self-help strategies, culminating in 24-hour emergency professional crisis support. When people struggle, they can lose the ability to generate and evaluate possible solutions. They may feel that their only option is to end their life. A Safety Plan provides a roadmap to safely navigate these feelings.

There are many Safety Plan templates freely available online, for example StayingSafe.net (Box 11.2).

Box 11.2 Using StayingSafe.net to make a Safety Plan

StayingSafe.net was co-produced by 4 Mental Health and their International Expert Reference Group, including people with lived experience, academics and practitioners, as a digital solution to equip people to make a Safety Plan. This website includes videos and detailed written guidance which makes it suitable for a person to make a Safety Plan on their own or with support from someone who is not a specialist. It has both a downloadable blank Safety Plan template for printing and completing as a hard copy, and an online Safety Plan for electronic completion and storage on a phone/mobile device. The online Safety Plan includes a range of 'tried and tested' strategies and ideas which are safe, evidence-informed and generated or reviewed by people with lived experience, ensuring that they are realistic and not patronising. It also includes free learning resources and free posters to download and print – ideal for waiting areas as well as clinical areas.

The following are some of the components of a Safety Plan that clinicians should consider when supporting people in distress, at risk of self-harm or suicide (Box 11.3). A Safety Plan comprises:

- Individualised self-help strategies/activities to instil hope
- Restriction of access to common means of suicide
- Activities to lift mood/calm/distract
- Contacts for social and emotional support
- Contacts for suicide prevention crisis support
- Professional support including crisis 24/7 (e.g. ED)

You do not have to be a mental health professional to support a patient to make a Safety Plan, although usually this is something that the liaison team will do when planning planning a safe discharge. Having a Safety Plan can empower a person to feel more confident that they can get through tough times. It can also remove some of the fear around recurrent suicidal thoughts or crises, for them and for their loved ones. It involves ensuring that if that a crisis or indeed the next crisis happens, a plan is in place to help the patient avoid suicide or harm, thus enabling a person to stay safe, even at 3 o'clock in the morning when they are struggling with suicidal thoughts.

Note that a Safety Plan does not replace treatment as usual or the need to refer to specialist mental health services.

A Safety Plan can be very useful in the ED or prehospital or medical ward setting. If a patient attends an ED with pneumonia, you may recommend admission with intravenous antibiotics. If this patient declines admission, then you would send that patient home with information and oral antibiotics. If a person with a Safety Plan attends the ED, it should be reviewed with the patient and steps taken to incorporate the Safety Plan into their management and treatment regime (as far as possible).

Box 11.3 Elements of a Safety Plan

Getting through right now
Strategies to 'get through right now' if overwhelmed:
- Reminders of hope and anything positive including 'inspirational quotes'
- Special photos: people, pets, special places
- 'Feel good' music to boost mood

Making your situation safer
- Remove anything that can be used for self-harm/suicide
- Avoid anything disinhibiting (e.g benzodiazepines/alcohol/drugs). Remove access to alcohol if not dependent, this may mean dispose or give to a friend to look after until the crisis is over
- Specific actions to remove, reduce or mitigate means for self-harm or suicide:
  - Remove medication from home during crisis period
  - Reduce medication, e.g. store most elsewhere, short scripts, dispense small amounts
  - Mitigate, e.g. locked box with key in different part of home or Safety Plan/special photo/card/letter stored with medication
- Consider whether safe alone/with someone and at home/ somewhere else

Things to lift or calm mood
- Activities to lift mood: anything enjoyable, e.g. connecting with some-one, thinking of positive future event/special memories, a special photo
- Activities to calm mood: meditation, yoga, accessing calming thoughts, e.g. special place or happy memory, journalling (write feelings in a diary or a letter)

Things to distract
- Thinking activities to 'take your mind away', e.g. listening to music, crosswords, Sudoku, TV, YouTube, films
- Doing activities to 'keep busy', e.g. exercise, cooking, art, chores, interacting with someone in person, via email, text or on social media

Sources of support
- Day-to-day support (not necessarily for discussing self-harm or suicide) from friends, family or people in your community especially if they help you feel better when you connect
- Try to include phone, text and messenger support, e.g. QWELL, KOOTH, Papyrus, Samaritans
- No need to tell the people on this list what you are going through or feeling

Specific support if distressed or thinking about self-harm or suicide
- One or two trusted, supportive confidants (friends, family, community members) and specialist helplines
- Prioritise the list and include multiple people/organisations in case a contact is unreachable
- If possible, it is better if supporters know and agree they are on a Safety Plan

Specific suicide and self-harm prevention
- 24-hour helplines or websites
- Local healthcare support and emergency NHS contact details for out of hours support

Introducing the Safety Plan at an appropriate early time will give hope and provide safe information to the patient even if they leave the department before the mental health team have reviewed or finalised their formal plan. It is the 'oral antibiotic' and may save their life.

A Safety Plan is evidenced-based and can help patients break the chain from suicidal thoughts or thoughts of harm to acting on those thoughts. It can remind the person of their personal strategies and contacts to help them reduce the level of distress.

Safety Plan templates and advice how to use can be downloaded free from the internet:

- https://www.stayingsafe.net/home: this is a good site to direct the patient to. It talks a patient through the process and explains why it is helpful. It is great for professionals as it has free learning resources (see Box 11.2)
- https://www.samaritans.org/how-we-can-help/if-youre-worried-about-someone-else/supporting-someone-suicidal-thoughts/creating-safety-plan/
- https://www.papyrus-uk.org

The following e-learning training modules are available from 4 Mental Health (https://lms.4mentalhealth.com):

- Suicide Awareness for Professionals
- Safety Planning

Figure 11.4 is a worked example of a Safety Plan.

My Safety Plan

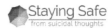Staying Safe
from suicidal thoughts

Getting through right now	List to Queen 'Don't stop me now', this was my first dance and it makes me smile Listen to classical music Stroke my cats Look at pictures of my wife/cats/friends Box breathing –meditation
Making my situation safer	Pass medications to friend Remove sharps –lock in shed and give my wife the key Inform those around me that I am struggling, e.g. close friends (inside and outside of work)
Things to lift or calm my mood	Play with the cats Listen to a comedy podcast/audiobook Watch comedy on Netflix/Prime Speak to Best man/friends/wife
Things to distract me	Play golf Spend time with friends Shoot things on X-box Spend time with godchildren Watch feel good movie
People to support me	Best man: Wife: Local friends: Oldest friends: Work colleagues/friends: Family:
Who I can talk to if I am distressed or thinking about self-harm or suicide	PAPYRUS HOPELINE247: 0800 068 4141 www.papyrus-uk.org Samaritans: 116 123 (24/7 www.samaritans.org) CALM: 0800 58 58 58 (5pm–midnight every day; support for men) Mind: 0300 123 3393 (9am–6pm Monday to Friday) QWELL: www.qwell.io Liverpool Light (crisis cafe): Liverpool Crisis Line: 0800 145 6570
Emergency professional support	My GP (family doctor): NHS Helpline England: 111 Emergency Department:

Figure 11.4 A worked example of a Safety Plan

PART 3

CHAPTER 12

Legal aspects of emergency psychiatry

Mental heath legislation and mental capacity legislation varies from country to country, and in some cases there are differences between counties or regions within a country. This will include legislation on deprivation of liberty, enforced care for the treatment of mental disorders, and the applications of capacity to consent to treatment. The information in this chapter is written in broad illustrative terms only, and does not reflect the law of any specific jurisdiction. Clinicians must refer to local policies and procedures, local training and applicable local laws in all subjects covered in this chapter. See also Limit of Liability/Disclaimer of Warranty on the title page verso.

Learning outcomes

After reading this chapter, you will be able to:

- List the major legal issues that arise in the assessment and management of psychiatric emergencies
- Describe the key components of each relevant legal issue
- Know where to find a more detailed and specific description of the legal frameworks in the jurisdiction where you work
- Identify the principles of maintaining patient confidentiality and the legal context
- Describe the importance of accurate and robust clinical documentation

Acute Psychiatric Emergencies: A Practical Approach, Second Edition.
Edited by Mark Buchanan and Damien Longson.
© 2025 John Wiley & Sons Ltd. Published 2025 by John Wiley & Sons Ltd.

12.1 Introduction

This chapter outlines the principles involved in the law as it applies to psychiatric emergencies. **The specifics of the legal frameworks for particular jurisdictions vary.** Summaries of the relevant law as it relates to the issues outlined in this chapter should be sought from your local training policies and procedures, and relevant online information.

The following sections outline the issues that are important when assessing and treating patients with a recognised mental disorder who are at risk to themselves or others.

12.2 Determining mental capacity

Mental capacity is a term that describes an individual's capability to make their own choices and decisions. Laws in different jurisdictions may vary.

If there is any doubt about whether the individual lacks capacity then an urgent second opinion should be sought. If doubt still remains, then an assumption should be made that they do have capacity and proceed on that basis. This means taking all reasonable steps to help them make their own decision.

The law may make a distinction between those who lack capacity as a result of an organic disorder such as epilepsy or brain injury, and those who lack capacity as a result of a mental illness.

Mental capacity assessment has a two-stage test:

1. The individual must meet the following criteria:
    - They understand the information given to them about treatment options and the necessity for treatment
    - They can retain information relevant to the treatment options
    - They can use or weigh up that information in coming to a decision
    - They can communicate that decision
2. A person must be suffering from a disturbance of the mind

> **Consider carefully whether the patient who is distressed, anxious, angry, depressed, bereaved or sleep-deprived has the capacity to weigh up the consequences of their actions.**
>
> **Consider joint capacity decisions with psychiatry in circumstances with potentially significant consequences to the patient.**

12.3   Treating a patient who does not have mental capacity

If you determine that someone lacks the capacity to decide about their treatment then the law may give you the opportunity to consider their best interests and act on this basis. Deciding on their best interests should lead you to consider:

- Whether the decision can wait until they regain capacity
- What the person has wanted in the past, and their relevant values and beliefs
- What their family and close friends say
- If you can involve the incapacitated person in the decision making

Deprivation of liberty

In many jurisdictions a person's freedom of movement cannot be limited without a court order, even if they lack capacity. In others, restrictions on movement can be authorised by other statutory organisations such as a local authority or a healthcare provider. Such restrictions are often limited in time and place.

Advance decisions and mental health

Some jurisdictions allow advance decisions to be made – terminology and their legal status will differ by jurisdiction. An **advance decision** is a statement of directions about what medical and healthcare treatment a patient wants to allow or refuse at a future time and the circumstances in which the decision will apply. These may apply only to physical health, mental health or both. Advance decisions may be stored with the patient's medical record and should be referred to if the patient has lost the capacity to make these decisions. The advance decision must be made when the patient has capacity and should be witnessed and signed. The patient must be an adult when making the advance decision.

Doctors may be able to override the advance decision if the patient is detained under mental health law, but this may only be for certain treatments, or where it is necessary to save life or prevent serious deterioration. Advance decisions about physical health treatments may remain valid even if the patient is detained under the law.

Other types of advanced statements or advanced directives may not be legal documents but provide information from the patient about their preferences on many matters, for example who to contact if they become unwell, who they would like to be kept informed and their preferences for treatment and medication. It does not have to be witnessed. You should take this into account when treating the patient, but it can be overridden, for example if there is a risk to the patient or others.

In the case of advance decisions and advance statements, if the patient has named an attorney under the law, and given them the power to make the same decisions or refusals, then they will make the decisions or refusals on the patient's behalf.

Detention for personal or public safety whilst in the community

If a person in the community is suspected of having a mental disorder and is thought to be in need of immediate care or treatment, or is thought to represent a risk to the safety of themselves or others, then it may be possible for them to be detained immediately under mental health laws. These powers may sit with the police (as powers of a police officer), with community health or mental health staff or with others. Generally, these powers will be powers of detention and will be limited in time and place (particularly making a distinction between a public and private space) and will be limited in what they allow to happen.

Following emergency detention, it will be specified what further legal routes may need to be pursued for ongoing detention (see following).

Stopping someone with a known or suspected mental health condition who is at risk of harm to self or others leaving the ED

The law will indicate whether or not you can take immediate steps to prevent someone lacking capacity leaving prior to a full assessment. Generally, any powers that are granted will be given to particular professionals, will be limited in time and must be proportionate.

If you think that the patient has a mental disorder and that their decision making is impaired because of this, that they need urgent investigations and treatment and/or they are a risk to themselves or others, then you will need to pursue legal routes to detain them in the Emergency Department (ED) if they still wish to leave. These legal routes differ in each jurisdiction and it is important to understand what actions you are able to take with each of these.

Sometimes, in an emergency situation, there is not enough time to seek judicial review. The law will be clear about who is empowered to prevent someone suspected of having severe mental illness from leaving before assessment, about how much force (if any) is allowed and about how long someone can be detained without formal assessment under mental health law.

Detention for assessment of psychiatric conditions in the ED under mental health laws

Although the law differs in different jurisdictions, emergency detention routes may only allow for assessment to decide if treatment is needed for a mental disorder. The patient would still need to consent to any treatment. If the patient refuses consent, then other detention routes should be considered.

Detention for treatment of psychiatric conditions in the ED under mental health laws

In England, there are no powers for the deprivation of liberty in the ED.

If treatment of the psychiatric condition is considered necessary and the patient refuses the treatment, then each jurisdiction will have detention options that permit the patient to be treated with or without their consent. Patients may have a right of appeal.

Detention for assessment and treatment of psychiatric conditions on the wards under mental health laws

There are generally legal powers that allow detention for diagnosis and, if necessary, treatment of psychiatric patients. These are different from the emergency powers. They may be differentiated by whether the patient has ever been assessed in hospital, has not been assessed in hospital for some time, or if they are well known to mental health teams and therefore further assessment is not required. Patients detained in this way will usually have the right to appeal. Different forms of detention exist with some only authorising specific treatments– for example emergency, but not regular, psychiatric treatment. In addition, some treatments, such as artificial nutrition or electroconvulsive therapy, may have additional legal safeguards and may not automatically be authorised.

Physical treatment of a patient detained under mental health laws

The law may differ in the area of consent depending on whether the proposed treatment is for mental or physical health needs. Laws under mental health acts often only apply to treatment for mental disorder. They may not apply to the treatment of physical disorders unless it is reasonable to say that the physical disorder is a symptom or an underlying cause of a mental disorder.

In some jurisdictions, doctors and nurses have the right to use holding powers where treatment for either a psychiatric or physical condition is deemed necessary and when a voluntary or informal patient (that is, a patient not currently detained under mental health laws) is wishing to leave. Generally, they must show that the patient must be immediately stopped from leaving for their own health or safety or for the protection of others. They must also show that the use of more formal legal routes would not be possible in the timeframe required. It is important to understand how this works within your own jurisdiction to ensure that you take the appropriate steps to work within the law.

12.4 Treating a patient who has mental capacity

> Consider carefully whether the patient who is distressed, anxious, angry, depressed, bereaved or sleep-deprived has the capacity to weigh up the consequences of their actions.
>
> Consider joint capacity decisions with psychiatry in circumstances with potentially significant consequences to the patient.

12.5 Consent

In general terms, if a patient has the capacity to consent, then their consent should be obtained prior to providing treatment. This consent should be informed consent and as outlined earlier you will need to assess the capacity of the patient to give this. Check the legal framework in your jurisdiction for details of express, implied or presumed consent and ensure that you fulfil the requirements with regard to obtaining this and documenting it.

For consent to be valid:
- **It must be given voluntarily**
- **There should be no duress**
- **The patient must have capacity**
- **Any information regarding risks, benefits, side effects and alternatives must be presented so that the patient can make an informed decision**
- **The patient must be able to communicate their choice**

12.6 Confidentiality

All healthcare practitioners have both a professional and a legal duty of confidentiality to their patients. Guidance and frameworks are produced by relevant professional bodies, employers and data protection legislation. These apply to all forms of records, not just those stored on computer media.

Consider confidentiality when providing a handover in the ED (Box 12.1). Avoid verbally presenting confidential information in the presence of relatives or anyone else without the patient's consent. Be particularly vigilant when passing information to colleagues via telephone, and remember that a curtain around a hospital bed does not prevent others hearing what is being said either to a patient or to colleagues.

Box 12.1 Important points in confidentiality

- Take all reasonable steps to keep a patient's information safe
- Obtain the patient's informed consent if you are passing on their information
- Only disclose identifiable information if it is absolutely necessary, and, when it is necessary, only disclose the minimum amount necessary
- Tell patients when you have disclosed their information

Source: Adapted from HCPC (2020).

12.7 Documentation

It is essential that accurate and robust clinical documentation is kept (Box 12.2). After any patient consultation – which may be either face-to-face, over the telephone or even when providing advice to a colleague – a record should be made either in writing or electronically in the patient's notes. It is also important to make accurate, signed, dated and timed records of discussions about the use of mental health legislation. There may well be particular procedures to follow and forms to be completed. Failure to make accurate records of these matters is not only potentially detrimental to patient care but may also render any deprivation of liberty unlawful or illegal.

Box 12.2 Clinical documentation

- Clinical documentation should be written in a clear, accurate and legible manner
- Record whether consent was obtained or not
- Detail all clinical findings, decisions made and actions taken
- Record the information given to patients
- Record any drugs prescribed or other investigation or treatment
- Identify whether confidential information has been shared

The most important factor is not when the notes were written, but what was recorded. Always strive to maintain the highest level of clinical documentation as this supports safe and effective patient care. This is not only a requirement of professional registration, but it may also help in your defence against complaint or allegation of poor practice.

12.8 Summary

The legal and professional frameworks covering consent, capacity, detention, confidentiality and documentation are an essential element in the management of patients. Clinicians should understand the principles of what these can achieve and the detail of the legal and professional frameworks within their own jurisdiction.

CHAPTER 13

Getting it right: non-technical skills

Learning outcomes

After reading this chapter, you will be able to:

- Explain why errors should be approached in a systemic way
- Describe how non-technical skills can improve the performance of individuals and teams in the healthcare environment to mitigate risks associated with adverse events

---

13.1   Introduction

Psychiatric emergencies are often high-pressure, evolving situations requiring good technical and clinical skills, but crucially also involving non-technical skills. Individuals from a variety of professional and specialty backgrounds come together and need to work effectively together if they are to prevent adverse events, manage the situation and ensure patient safety.

This chapter provides a brief introduction to some of the non-technical skills that can improve the performance of individuals and teams in the healthcare environment.

13.2   Errors in the healthcare setting

Consider this example of an adverse event.

> A patient is brought to the Emergency Department (ED) with a self-inflicted wound. Three hours later the patient is found cyanosed with a neck ligature tied round a coat hook, in one of the assessment rooms. What are the potential causes of this situation (Table 13.1)?

Acute Psychiatric Emergencies: A Practical Approach, Second Edition.
Edited by Mark Buchanan and Damien Longson.
© 2025 John Wiley & Sons Ltd. Published 2025 by John Wiley & Sons Ltd.

Table 13.1 Potential causes of our example error	
Cause	**Error type**
The triage nurse was very busy and did not complete a risk assessment	Initial assessment delay
The room used was inappropriately designed with non-collapsible hooks	Environmental error
The ED policy did not stipulate that any self-harm should receive immediate parallel mental health risk assessment	Policy error
The unit was short-staffed and there was no nurse overseeing that area	Supervision error
The ED doctor who assessed the patient did not ask any questions about future intent	Assessment error
The ligature cutter was not always kept in the same place and could not be found	Equipment error
None of the individuals involved so far had shared information about risk concerns	Communication error
No-one had written an observation plan for this patient	Management plan failure

However many checks and procedures are put in place, errors will still occur and may cause harm to patients. It is vital therefore that we look to work in a way that, wherever possible, reduces the occurrence of errors and ensures that when they do occur this minimises the chance of it resulting in an adverse event.

Reason's taxonomy of errors (Figure 13.1) illustrates how errors can be described as sharp (within clinical practice) and blunt (within the wider system).

Blunt end
Design phase

Sharp end
Clinical practice

Decreasing time to think

Issue with
Policies,
procedures, design
infrastructure,
building layout etc

Error types
Mistakes, slips,
lapses, rule-based
errors, knowledge-
based errors

Figure 13.1 Reason's taxonomy of errors

Because errors are multifactorial, it is typically found that organisational or blunt issues often coexist with clinical or sharp errors; in fact it is rare for an isolated error to occur. It is not uncommon for there to be a chain of events that results in the adverse event. The 'Swiss cheese model' demonstrates how apparently random, unconnected incidents and organisational decisions can collectively increase the likelihood of an adverse event (Figure 13.2). Conversely, a standardised system with good defences can capture these errors and prevent adverse events.

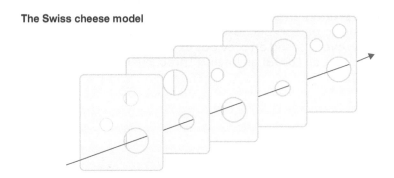

The Swiss cheese model

Figure 13.2 The Swiss cheese model

Each of the slices of Swiss cheese represents barriers which, under ideal circumstances, would prevent or detect the error. The holes represent weaknesses in these barriers; if the holes align, the error passes through undetected.

Reconsider the earlier example using the Swiss cheese model.

The first slice is the hospital's policies and procedures, and the structural design of the ED. The second slice is the staffing levels, and the resourcing of the department. The third slice is the availability of mental health expertise in the department. The fourth slice is the risk assessment skills of the individuals involved. The final slice is compliance oversight of standard procedures, such as where to keep safety equipment.

In this example, there were large holes in each slice, and some slices were missing altogether. The end result was that multiple defences were weakened or removed and error was more likely, and the error was more likely to cause harm.

There are two views on human errors:

- The first sees human errors as the causal factors in adverse events. This perspective will tend to blame individuals and lead to a punitive culture
- The second sees errors as the symptoms of systemic failure. This perspective will tend to blame individuals less and look for broader issues

When an adverse event occurs, a systemic approach should be used to understand it. However, general it takes several months to work on and improve systemic issues. In the interval, improving clinicians' non-technical skills can help to prevent adverse events.

13.3   Situation awareness

Situation awareness is a phrase used to describe an overall awareness and understanding of a situation in terms of what we are experiencing and what we predict may happen. It involves gathering information through all the senses, and interpreting this information. Situation awareness inevitably differs from person to person because the human brain selectively attends to aspects of a new event based on previous experiences. Situation awareness is described by Flin et al. (2008) as having three levels which build on each other (Figure 13.3).

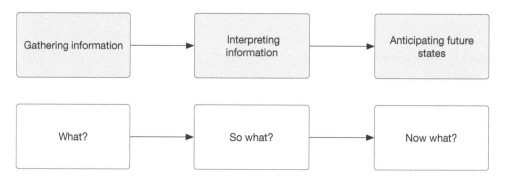

Figure 13.3 Situation awareness

Level one: gathering information

Information is routinely gathered through all of our senses. Some of it we attend to consciously, some unconsciously. In an acute mental health emergency, what we see and what we hear are the key ways in which we gather information. However, both are prone to significant errors: what we **think** we saw or heard may not be correct; our senses may let us down; or our immediate recall may be inaccurate. For example, it is important to really concentrate on seeing what is actually there. Figure 13.4 shows the similar package design of two different medications, making errors more likely.

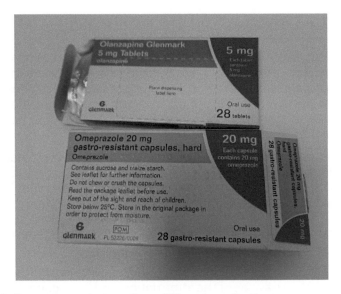

Figure 13.4 Similar package design of two different medications

Level two: interpreting information

This is the point at which data (what we see, hear, smell, etc.) are processed in order to make sense of the current situation. Everyone's capacity to interpret and understand a situation is dependent on the information they have gathered. In addition to this filter, new events are interpreted, or made sense of, through the prism of prior learning that has been stored in long-term memory. This is sometimes described as an individual's mental model. If these mental models are partial, vague or poorly anchored in memory, it is harder to make sense of what is happening in the moment, and therefore there is an increased risk of faulty comprehension and ultimately unsafe decision making. In order to mitigate this risk, it is helpful to seek out other peoples' mental models; this can be a simple and effective way of increasing safety and making better decisions.

Level three: anticipating future states

Level three builds on the analysis that was a key component of the second level as the practitioner considers what might happen next. In a dynamic setting, such as a consultation with someone who is acutely disturbed, it is important to remain vigilant to changes in what is happening and to have more than one planned response and be able to make rapid and safe adaptations. Learning to predict the effects of particular interventions is a key element of the APEx course. Remaining open to the unexpected is, however, essential.

It is only after thinking through each of these three steps that someone will be able to make a decision.

13.4 Decision making

On the face of it, the practice of decision making is familiar to everyone. To make a good decision a person needs to assess all aspects of a problem, identify the possible responses, consider the consequences of each of those responses and then weigh up the advantages and disadvantages. Having completed this analysis, they then need to communicate their decision to the patient and to their team.

Good situation awareness as described earlier (what, so what, now what) is a prerequisite to sound decision making. The clinician must ensure they have all the key information. Everyone involved in the situation should be on the alert for ambiguities or conflicting information and be ready to share their own mental model to check it does not differ from that of others. Any inconsistent facts should be treated as potential markers for defective situation awareness. They should never be brushed off as unimportant anomalies.

When there are no time pressures, a decision should not be made until the team is satisfied they have all of the information and have considered all of the options. Where time is an issue, a certain amount of pragmatism must be employed. There is plenty of evidence to confirm that practice and experience can mitigate some of the negative effects of abbreviating a decision-making process. However, those making decisions under such circumstances need to note the short-cuts they have taken. They should be ready to receive feedback from those around them, particularly if anyone has significant concerns about the proposed course of action.

13.5 Cognitive bias

Good decision making in an acute mental health emergency can be compromised by cognitive bias, in particular anchoring bias, confirmation bias and diagnostic overshadowing. We will look at these through an examination of a case.

> John attends the ED agitated and hallucinating. The paramedics state that he has previously been known to be alcohol dependent. His symptoms are attributed to alcohol withdrawal. He deteriorates and has a large seizure. It is thought that this is alcohol withdrawal related. He is observed for an hour and as his level of consciousness does not improve he is taken for a CT scan. The scan shows a large bleed. Subsequent history from John's family is that he has been sober for 3 months after rehab.

Anchoring bias

This bias represents a common cognitive error, whereby all subsequent information about a scenario is viewed through the prism of the earliest information encountered (Tversky and Kahneman, 1974). This has been observed even when the anchoring information is irrelevant or incorrect (Figure 13.5). When asked, for example, to predict how tall a tree is, people will give a higher estimate if they have just been made to think about a high number, and a lower estimate if they have just been made to think about a lower number.

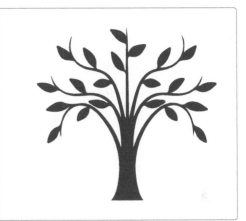

Is the tree taller than 90 metres?

How tall is the tree?

Is the tree taller than 20 metres?

How tall is the tree?

When asked, people will be subconsciously influenced by the number they were first given which is why this bias is known as anchoring bias.

Figure 13.5 Anchoring bias

Anchoring bias means, for example, that teams can misinterpret clinical signs or test results based on a false initial assumption about their diagnosis. This is a particular problem with organic causes of disturbing behaviour as with John's case. The anchor there was the mention of alcohol dependence.

Confirmation bias

Confirmation bias occurs when the wrong model is being applied to a situation and facts are then interpreted to fit with this model. Cues that might not support the model are ignored, rejected or dismissed as irrelevant/inaccurate. This bias describes the tendency for people to seek confirming rather than disconfirming information. An easy trap to fall into is presenting a problem to someone in a way that expects them to agree with what one has said. This is likely to lead to confirmation bias. There is value in seeking opinions from those who you know might have a different perspective. It is also good practice to gather a number of opinions, to remain open to being challenged and to challenge others even when they are senior.

Going back to John – he is alcohol dependent, and patients with alcohol dependence are known to have seizures. When he presents with a seizure as described, the seizure (a fact) is made to fit the model (patients with alcohol dependence have fits). The seizure is attributed to alcohol withdrawal due to confirmation bias.

Diagnostic overshadowing

Diagnostic overshadowing arises when a patient's presentation or symptoms are attributed to a pre-existing (and maybe also apparent) mental health condition, rather than fully exploring all the historical and acute factors.

Completing assessments in full, using structured approaches such as ABCD/AEIO and PHRASED, even when the situation may seem clear, is one way to prevent diagnostic overshadowing.

These cognitive biases might seem trivial or easily avoided but vulnerability to them is universal, and people vastly overestimate their ability to notice critical events when under pressure.

Decision making is known to be degraded at times of high workload, and these and other biasing effects can be significant. Taking a short time out can make individuals' and teams' responses more efficient by reducing errors of fixation and time wasted on unnecessary or low-priority tasks. On the APEx course, clinicians are encouraged to take mini time-outs to re-evaluate, seek wider views and consider potential options.

13.6   Communication

Psychiatric emergencies are often unfamiliar or frightening for the patient, other patients in the department and for the staff involved. Whether the situation is an urgent one, such as rapid tranquillisation, or less immediate, such as a more slowly unfolding emergency, good communication is essential for a positive outcome.

Directed communication

When communicating face-to-face, in an acute setting, a message is often announced to a room where nobody acknowledges it. Targeting our communications towards specified individuals in what is sometimes referred to as 'directed communication' is now seen to be an essential element in improving communication. Most often this means using a person's name, but can mean using their role if their name is unknown.

If an untargeted instruction is offered to a group, for example 'Can someone bring me the rapid tranquillisation kit', then there is a chance that everyone in the room will assume that someone else is going to perform the task. Compare this with: 'Seema, can you bring me the rapid tranquillisation kit'; now it becomes Seema's responsibility and she will do it.

The second reason for using someone's name in directed communication relates to how the brain processes auditory information. Environmental sounds are subconsciously monitored; the likelihood of information passing from the subconscious to the conscious mind depends on several factors. The amount of cognitive capacity a person has at a given time is limited, and salience (or how personally relevant it is) has an impact. Even when you are concentrating hard on one task or conversation, you will hear your own name.

Briefing and handover

Our mental models are affected by our previous experiences but also by the information/briefing that we received before the event. A good pre-brief will positively influence how the team frame the situation and which mental models they draw on. Where a briefing is accurate it is extremely helpful; where it is inaccurate, because it influences how we interpret information, it can lead to errors. We are more likely to fit what we see to what we expect to see (confirmation bias) and therefore make inaccurate conclusions. Practising good briefings and handovers is time well spent.

There are a variety of tools, such as SBAR (situation, background, assessment and recommendation), which facilitate planning and organising a message, making it succinct and focused. A good SBAR provides a handover in a logical and expected order. It is also a tool of empowerment allowing the sender (who may be more junior) to request an action from a more senior individual.

Effective communication with a feedback loop

Errors can occur at any level or multiple levels. Remember our earlier scenario of a busy clinical situation where the patient presented following self-harm. The triage nurse moved the patient into a room and assumed that the staff in that area would continue the care from there. Whose job was it to ensure communication had happened? Consider how much better the outcome would have been if the following simple communication and feedback loop had occurred:

> Triage nurse to supervising nurse: *'I've just put Mr X into the blue room. He is at high risk of further self-harm, so I think he needs to have someone with him at all times'*

> Supervising nurse to triage nurse: *'OK – Mr X is in the blue room. I'll arrange for him to have someone with him at all times, and I'll ask the mental health team to assess him straight away'*

We now know that the message has been transmitted and received correctly (Figure 13.6).

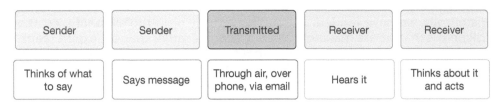

Figure 13.6 Elements of communication

For this process to work, both parties (the sender and receiver) need to understand and expect it – again demonstrating the need to practise and train together.

Communicating well with patients

In psychiatric emergencies much of the assessment is carried out by communicating with the patient or those accompanying them; there are generally few physical tests to carry out, or signs to elicit. In many cases there will be barriers to communication, such as language, cultural norms or disturbed behaviour. Preconceptions of what is and is not 'normal' may affect the assessment, leading to bias at best, and poor care with prejudice at worst. To avoid these, consider the following (Figure 13.7).

DO

- Seek as much information from those around you as possible, especially before they leave the department.

- Identify if there is anyone around who can help with communication difficulties

- Check available records to see if they supplement the information available

- Escalate concerns about communication as soon as possible

DO NOT

- Pigeonhole patients into characteristic groups

- Delay decision-making in emergency situations

- Overreact – many situations can wait until more information is available, especially when communication is difficult.

Figure 13.7 Avoiding preconceptions

13.7 Managing critical situations

Historically, we have tended to train individually or in professional silos; the risk here is that we are making a 'team of experts' rather than an 'expert team'. The APEx course is fundamentally about working across traditional clinical areas, and will give the opportunity to practise this.

Leadership

The leader's role is multifaceted and includes directing the team, assigning tasks and assessing performance, motivating and encouraging the team to work together, and planning and organising. Perhaps most significantly in the context of acute mental health emergencies, the leader's key role is to ensure that everyone remains safe, and throughout this book the emphasis on the Unified assessment is driven by this imperative.

All leadership skills and behaviours need to be developed and practised. There are different leadership styles that can be categorised as delegating, consulting, coaching, facilitating and directing. Effective leaders are able to choose the most appropriate style for the situation they are facing. For example, if there is a junior present who needs to practise a specific skill then coaching is appropriate. If a patient suddenly becomes violent then the leader needs to make a rapid decision and direct others as to what to do.

Hierarchy

Within the team there needs to be a hierarchy. The leader is at the top of this as the person coordinating the situation, directing and making the decisions. However, this should not be absolute. Where the hierarchical gradient is too steep, the leader is in a position in which their decisions are beyond question and the followers blindly follow their orders. This is not safe because leaders are humans too and also make errors: their team is their safety net.

Safe practice is achieved where the followers feel they can raise concerns or question instructions. This must always be understood by the leaders as much as the followers. One way to reduce the hierarchy is for the leader to invite the team's thoughts and concerns particularly around patient safety issues. This in itself will lead to improved patient care.

Raising concerns

It is important to learn how to raise concerns appropriately. One method that is sometimes used to raise concerns is PACE (probing, alerting, challenging or declaring an emergency (Figure 13.8)).

PACE

Stage		Level of concern
P	Probe	I think you need to know what is happening
A	Alert	I think something bad might happen
C	Challenge	I know something bad will happen
E	Emergency	I will not let it happen

Figure 13.8 PACE

Consider the evolving situation below, involving one of the healthcare assistants (HCAs) in the ED who has noticed Mr X in a side room, on his own. How would the patient's outcome have been altered if the HCA carried out the PACE protocol?

	The HCA thinks	The HCA says to the nurse in charge
Probe – this is used where a person notices something they think might be a problem. They verbalise the issue, often as a question	That person seems distressed	'Have you noticed that Mr X seems quite upset?'
Alert – the observer strengthens and directs their statement and suggests a course of action	Mr X seems to have found some tubigrip	'Mr X has found some tubigrip. I don't think that room is safe, and I think he needs observation'
Challenge – the situation requires urgent attention. One of the key protagonists needs to be directly engaged. If possible the speaker places themselves into the eye line of the person they wish to communicate with	Mr X is on his own, in an unsafe room, with a ligature	'You must go in to see Mr X now – I am worried for his safety'
Emergency – this is used where all else has failed and/or the observer perceives a critical event is about to occur. Where possible a physical signal or physical barrier should be employed together with clear verbalisation	No one is doing anything	'I am taking control of this situation. I have asked Rishi to sit in with Mr X until the situation is made safe'

The PACE structure can be commenced at any appropriate level and escalated until a satisfactory response is gained. If an adverse event is imminent then it may be relevant to start at the 'declaring emergency' stage, whereas a much lower level of concern may well start at a 'probing' question.

13.8   Preventing errors

Situations when errors are more likely

If we are aware that errors are more likely we can be more proactive in detecting them. Two common situations that increase the likelihood of errors are stress and fatigue. Stress is not only a source of error when we are overworked and overstimulated, but also at the other end of the spectrum when we are understimulated we become inattentive.

The acronym **I'M SAFE** (Figure 13.9) has been used to describe situations when errors are more likely:

I'M SAFE

Stage		Level of concern
I	Illness	Is the health carer suffering from any illness or symptom of an illness which might affect them?
M	Medications	Is the health carer currently taking any drugs that might affect them?
S	Stress	Is the health carer overly worried about other factors in their life?
A	Alcohol	Although the health carer should not be under alcohol influence at work, they also should consider their alcohol consumption within the last 8 to 24 hours.
F	Fatigue	Has the health carer had sufficient sleep and adequate nutrition?
E	Emotion	Has the health carer fully recovered from any extremely upsetting events such as the loss of a family member?

Figure 13.9 I'M SAFE

Ideally, individuals who are potentially compromised need to be supported appropriately, allowed time to recover and the team made aware. How this can be achieved in the middle of a night shift though can be problematic.

Distractions

Errors are also more likely to occur when clinicians are distracted. Within healthcare settings distractions are the norm to such an extent individuals are often not even aware of them. On a daily basis we are distracted by our phones, bleeps and computers; by people talking to us; and by interruptions outside our control. The risk is that the moment of the distraction leads to a crucial mistake or information being missed. In a psychiatric setting, this may alter the flow of a structured risk assessment, leading to missed components and an incorrect conclusion. From a safety perspective it might lead to a dangerous implement being unveiled. When doing critical tasks, such as taking a history from a patient in an acute mental health crisis, it is important to try to prevent and challenge interruptions.

Cognitive aids: checklists, guidelines and protocols

Cognitive aids such as guidelines, mnemonics and algorithms are useful because the human memory is not infallible. They also confer team understanding through the use of a standardised response. This reduces stress. This is especially true where an uncommon emergency event occurs. The team may be unfamiliar with one another and each member will be trying to remember what to do, what treatments are required and in what order. Using the relevant cognitive aid as a prompt means that everyone involved in the care of the patient is following the same pathway and can plan ahead.

Calling for help early

Trainee staff are often reluctant to call for senior help, partly due to not recognising the severity of the situation and also due to concerns about wasting the time of seniors. With all emergency events, appropriate help should be summoned as soon as possible. In the case of an escalating crisis with an acutely disturbed patient it can be essential to call for help in the form of security personnel, or simply more bodies to assist with managing and/or restraining someone who risks being a danger to themselves or others. Help may not arrive instantly and it is important not to put yourself at risk while waiting for others.

Mutual support and task assistance

Assisting others in tasks contributes to the development of a robust and trustworthy team. Essential strategies for this include:

- Cultivating psychological safety and shielding one another from excessive work demands
- Framing all offers and requests for help within the context of patient safety
- Nurturing an environment where seeking and offering assistance is the norm
- Demonstrating a willingness to seek help and taking responsibility for tackling challenges and finding solutions
- Engaging in reciprocal assistance with patients and family caregivers

Team resilience is bolstered by a simple enquiry to fellow team members, '*I have 10 minutes. How can I be of assistance?*'

Debriefing

Wherever possible a debrief should be facilitated following critical events, even if brief, as this encourages healthcare professionals to normalise talking about difficult situations. A debrief immediately after an event is described as a 'hot' debrief and it has the aim of ensuring psychological safety. There is a place for this at the end of a shift or difficult emergency to ensure that staff are OK as they go home. The 'hot' debrief is not about learning points or establishing what happened. That can wait for the 'cold' debrief, days or even weeks after the event. This is usually facilitated by a trained individual with the intention of learning from the event and providing pointers moving forwards.

It is best practice to debrief after engaging in restraint or rapid tranquillisation.

13.9   Summary

This chapter has given a brief introduction to the clinical human factors and non-technical skills that are relevant to acute mental health emergencies.

These situations, which are initially critical, sometimes become greatly extended moments requiring resilience from staff. They sometimes lead to poor team working, patient harm and adverse events. It is crucial to use every opportunity to reflect and develop your own performance and influence the development of those around you.

It is important to pre-empt possible risks, think about how biases can affect the way we approach and manage the patient attending in crisis, and consider how outside influences can affect how we perform.

The patient experience

Learning outcomes

After reading this chapter, you will be able to:

- Recognise the experience of attending the Emergency Department with a mental health crisis from the perspective of a patient
- Identify potential improvements to optimise the patient experience

---

14.1   Introduction

This chapter is based on an interview with a patient who has had experience of personal mental health crises and of mental health crises within her family.

The themes that emerged during the interview are:

- Emotional safety
- Balance of care between physical and mental health
- Attitudes and responses of staff
- Privacy and confidentiality
- Communication with patient, parent and carer
- Environmental issues

Each of these is covered in more detail here.

14.2   Aspects of a patient's experience

Emotional safety

Emotional safety is often ignored, with a focus purely on physical safety. Emergency medicine staff can improve emotional safety by talking to the patient and providing a 'reassuring touch'. Once physical safety is assured,

---

Acute Psychiatric Emergencies: A Practical Approach, Second Edition.
Edited by Mark Buchanan and Damien Longson.
© 2025 John Wiley & Sons Ltd. Published 2025 by John Wiley & Sons Ltd.

emotional safety should be the focus, with attention paid to making sure that the environment does not feel hostile in any way. This can be supported by consideration of the areas covered elsewhere within this chapter such as attitudes and responses of staff, balance of care and communication.

Balance of care

The balance between physical and emotional care for those with a mental health crisis can be variable. In some situations, mental health patients present with a combination of physical and mental health issues; in others, the presentation requires no physical treatment. It is important in the emergency medicine setting to consider the point at which the emergency medicine team care of the patient begins and ends. Just dealing with the physical issue and not focusing on emotional safety may result in the underlying problem being ignored. The patient may then reattend repeatedly seeking the emotional support that they need.

Even in situations where there is a decision taken that further support is required from the psychiatry team, experience has shown that there is a tendency for the emergency medicine staff to 'step back' while waiting for the psychiatry team to arrive. Verbal interactions, in addition to physical monitoring checks, could make a difference in this situation, with the patient then feeling supported during the transition from the care of the emergency medicine team to the psychiatry team. This is also the case where someone is detained in the department but no physical health checks are required, when some level of interaction would make patients not feel 'abandoned' by the emergency medicine team.

A better balance between the questions asked by the emergency medicine team and the psychiatry team can reduce distressing repetition. Consider what it is essential to know now and what can wait until the full psychosocial assessment.

The wait for the psychosocial assessment can be distressing for the patient and their family. This is particularly so if this involves lengthy waits in the Emergency Department (ED) or admission overnight into a hospital bed.

It is important to consider how often patients should be monitored and document at least the level of distress and any interventions that have been needed. This may include what has worked and what has not, this includes de-escalation and medication.

Attitudes and responses of staff

The attitude of staff can make attendance in the department a daunting experience for mental health patients. Experience of 'eye-rolling' and comments such as '*Oh it's you again*' can make patients feel less deserving of care. Comments like '*It's not as bad as last time*' while intended to be reassuring can have unexpected consequences on someone who is a repeat attendee with self-harm. On one occasion a comment like that resulted in the patient '*going into the hospital toilet and making the cut bigger*' so that she 'deserved' the care she needed.

It only needs one person to be perceived as having this attitude to lead to a 'negative pathway'. It can, potentially, prompt someone to leave the department before a full psychosocial assessment.

Comments which were in all likelihood not intended to be negative or derogatory, such as '*Why do you keep doing this to your beautiful arms*', can be taken as such by someone who is vulnerable with low self-esteem, low self-confidence and low self-worth. They hear: '*You're a rubbish person, you're thoughtless*'.

Comments that dismiss the level of distress someone is in, such as '*You're not going to be silly again are you*' may be heard in a different way than intended. Patients hear '*You are behaving badly*' and '*You may be punished*'.

It is important to ensure there is a culture in your service that challenges stigma; to not challenge condones these attitudes. It may mean discussing with your team leaders or managers and asking them to deal with this.

Privacy and confidentiality

In cubicles, in particular, privacy can be an issue with only the curtain separating the patient from other patients and 'common' areas. The sensitive nature of conversations about mental health issues should be considered. Concerns that they may be overheard may make the patient reluctant to be open and this can then be a barrier to their ongoing treatment.

In addition, consideration should be given to the impact on the patient of physical signals that make their situation less private, such as being flanked by police officers or security guards whilst walking through a hospital if they are being detained for their own safety. Consideration of their safety, but also other approaches to this, may mean that the escort is less obvious. Provision of a side room whilst waiting for admission to a ward, rather than waiting with the escort in public areas, may also make their situation more private.

Communication

Regular communication with the patient themselves and, in the case of children, with them and their parent/carer can often be forgotten if the patient has been 'handed over' to the psychiatry team and the ED staff are waiting for them to arrive. The delays can often be considerable and during this period regular updates are important to provide support and reassurance.

Often families are not aware of the steps involved in arranging a psychosocial assessment, and an explanation of this and what the assessment will involve can make the situation feel more controlled. Briefing the family, where confidentiality permits, before they see their loved one, can prepare them and make the initial meeting more manageable and less stressful for them and the patient.

The patient themselves can be 'scared', 'distressed' and 'anxious' about what is happening to them and about what the reactions of their family will be when they arrive. This can further heighten their feelings and emotions, and communicating with them regularly and reassuring them can help alleviate this.

Being honest and open about timeframes can also mean that family members can go for food, drink and respite breaks.

Environmental issues

In the ED, guideline changes over recent years have resulted in improvements to the physical environment for mental health patients. From an emotional perspective, however, it is often not the best environment. A cubicle with a surrounding curtain can be 'claustrophobic and scary' and voices can be heard from all around which can be 'disorientating'. For someone who is intent on self-harm, these environments may be safer, but they are not completely safe and regular checks should be made and can help to make the patient calmer and emotionally safer.

Rooms that are set up for the physical safety of someone who is being detained for their own safety can be like 'goldfish bowls' with the patient feeling watched. Also, with nothing available that can be a risk to the patient they can be *'boring'*, with nothing to keep patients occupied during their wait.

Other environmental issues to consider during a wait for the psychiatry team are food, drink, toilet and, in some cases, cigarette breaks. Again, this supports calmer and emotionally safer patient experiences.

14.3 Summary

From a patient perspective, there are many small, but essential, changes that can be made that would improve their experience of attending an ED with a mental health crisis and would support their ongoing emotional safety.

Working group for second edition

Roger Alcock MBChB, BSc(Hons), FRCP Edin, DCH, FRCEM, FRGS, Consultant in Emergency Medicine and Paediatric Emergency Medicine, Victoria Hospital, NHS Fife

David Baden PhD, Emergency Physician, Diakonessenhuis Utrecht; President of the Dutch Society of Emergency Physicians (DSEP)

Mark Buchanan FCEM, Consultant in Adult and Paediatric Emergency Medicine, Arrowe Park Hospital, Wirral University Teaching Hospital NHS Trust; Honorary Clinical Senior Lecturer, University of Liverpool

Rebecca Chubb MRCPsych, Locum Consultant Psychiatrist, North Staffordshire Combined Healthcare NHS Trust

Vanessa Craig MB, BCh, BAO, MRCPsych, Consultant Liaison Psychiatrist, Manchester Royal Infirmary, Greater Manchester Health HNS Foundation Trust; Honorary Senior Lecturer in Medical Education, School of Medical Sciences, University of Manchester

Sandrine Dénéréaz Paramedic, Master in Public Administration, Paramedic School Director, Lausanne, Switzerland

Fiona Donnelly BSc, MBChB, MRCPsych, PgDip Psychiatry, PGDip Health and Public Leadership, Consultant Psychiatrist, Mental Health and Home Treatment Team, Wythenshawe Hospital

James Ferguson FRCSEd, FRCS(A&E), FRCEM, FRCPE, FRSM, Consultant Surgeon in Emergency Medicine, NHS Grampian

Elspeth Guthrie MBChB, MSc, MD, FRCPsych, Professor of Psychological Medicine, Leeds Institute of Health Sciences, University of Leeds

Damien Longson PhD, FRCPsych, Consultant Liaison Psychiatrist, Greater Manchester Mental Health NHS Foundation Trust; Honorary Professor of Psychiatry, University of Manchester

Aaron McMeekin MBChB, LLB(Hons), MSc(Oxon), MRCPsych, PGCertMedEd, FHEA, Consultant Perinatal Psychiatrist, Greater Manchester Mental Health NHS Foundation Trust; Honorary Senior Clinical Teacher, Academic Unit of Medical Education, University of Sheffield

Andrew M. Russell MBChB, MRCS, FRCEM, Consultant in Emergency Medicine, University Hospital Monklands, Lanarkshire

Murray Smith MRCPsych, Consultant Liaison Psychiatrist, Department of Psychological Medicine, Aberdeen Royal Infirmary, NHS Grampian

Working group for first edition

Roger Alcock MB, ChB, BSc(hons), FRCP Edin, DCH, FRCEM, Consultant in Emergency Medicine and Paediatric Emergency Medicine, Forth Valley Royal Hospital, Larbert

Helen Bradford MA, DClinPsy, CPsychol, AFBPsS, Consultant Clinical Psychologist, Bradford Psychology

Mark Buchanan Consultant in Adult and Paediatric Emergency Medicine, Arrowe Park Hospital

Vanessa Craig MBBCh, BAO, MRCPsych, Consultant Liaison Psychiatrist, Greater Manchester Mental Health NHS Foundation Trust, Manchester Royal Infirmary

Sandrine Dénéréaz Paramedic – Paramedics School Director, École Supérieure d'Ambulancier et Soins d'Urgence Romande, Lausanne, Switzerland; President, Commission for Emergencies Health Measures, Lausanne

Fiona Donnelly BSc, MBChB, MRCPsych, PgDip Psychiatry, PGDip Health and Public Leadership, Consultant Psychiatrist, Mental Health and Home Treatment Team, Wythenshawe Hospital

James Ferguson MBChB, FRCSEd, FRCS(A&E), FRCEM, FRCPE, Professor in Remote Medicine, Robert Gordon University; Reader in Emergency Medicine, Aberdeen University; Clinical Lead, Scottish Centre for Telehealth and Telecare and Digital Health and Care Institute

Sarah Gaskell DClinPsy, PGDip, Consultant Clinical Psychologist, Head of Paediatric Psychosocial Services, Royal Manchester Children's Hospital

Elspeth Guthrie MBChB, MSc, MD, FRCPsych, Professor of Psychological Medicine, Leeds Institute of Health Sciences, University of Leeds

Damien Longson PhD, FRCPsych, Consultant Liaison Psychiatrist, Greater Manchester Foundation Trust; Associate Dean, Royal College of Psychiatrists

Kevin Mackway-Jones MA, DH, FRCP, FRCS, FRCEM, Professor of Emergency Medicine, Manchester Royal Infirmary and the Royal Manchester Children's Hospital; Director of Postgraduate Medicine, Manchester Metropolitan University

Laura McGregor FRCEM, MRCP, DTMH, DIMC, Consultant in Emergency Medicine, University Hospital Monklands; Educational Coordinator, Emergency Medicine, Scottish Centre for Simulation and Clinical Human Factors

Aaron McMeekin MBChB, LLB(Hons), MSc(Oxon), MRCPsych, PGCertMedEd, FHEA, Consultant Perinatal Psychiatrist, Greater Manchester Mental Health NHS Foundation Trust; Honorary Lecturer, Academic Unit of Medical Education, University of Sheffield

Andrew McNeill Russell MBChB, MRCS, FRCEM, Consultant in Emergency Medicine, University Hospital Monklands

Rachel Thomasson PhD, MRCPsych, Consultant Neuropsychiatrist, Manchester Centre for Clinical Neurosciences, Salford Royal NHS Foundation Trust

Sue Wieteska CEO, Advanced Life Support Group

Damian Wood MBChB, DCH, MRCPCH, Consultant Paediatrician, Nottingham Children's Hospital, Queen's Medical Centre

Contributors to first edition

Helen Bradford MA, DClinPsy, CPsychol, AFBPsS, Consultant Clinical Psychologist, Bradford Psychology

Fiona Donnelly BSc, MBChB, MRCPsych, PGDip Psychiatry, PGDip Health and Public Leadership, Consultant Psychiatrist, Mental Health and Home Treatment Team, Wythenshawe Hospital

Richard J. Drake BSc, MBChB, MRCPsych, PhD, Clinical Lead for Mental Health, Health Innovation Manchester; Honorary Consultant, Greater Manchester Mental Health NHS Foundation Trust; Senior Lecturer, Division of Psychology and Mental Health, School of Health Sciences, Faculty of Biology, Medicine and Health, University of Manchester

Peter-Marc Fortune FRCPCH, FFICM, FAcadMEd, Consultant Paediatric Intensivist, Associate Medical Director, Royal Manchester Children's Hospital

Elspeth Guthrie MBChB, MSc, MD, FRCPsych, Professor of Psychological Medicine, Leeds Institute of Health Services, University of Leeds

Mark Hellaby MSc, Med, PG Cert, BSc(Hons) RODP, FHEA, North West Simulation Education Network Manager, NHS Health Education England

Damien Longson PhD, FRCPsych, Consultant Liaison Psychiatrist, Greater Manchester Foundation Trust; Associate Dean, Royal College of Psychiatrists

Kevin Mackway-Jones MA, DH, FRCP, FRCS, FRCEM, Professor of Emergency Medicine, Manchester Royal Infirmary and the Royal Manchester Children's Hospital; Director of Postgraduate Medicine, Manchester Metropolitan University

Aaron McMeekin MBChB, LLB(Hons), MSc(Oxon), MRCPsych, PGCertMedEd, FHEA, Consultant Perinatal Psychiatrist, Greater Manchester Mental Health NHS Foundation Trust; Honorary Lecturer, Academic Unit of Medical Education, University of Sheffield

Rachel Thomasson PhD, MRCPsych, Consultant Neuropsychiatrist, Manchester Centre for Clinical Neurosciences, Salford Royal NHS Foundation Trust

References and further reading

Chapter 1

NHS England (2016). *Achieving Better Access to 24/7 Urgent and Emergency Mental Health Care – Part 2: Implementing the Evidence-based Treatment Pathway for Urgent and Emergency Liaison Mental Health Services for Adults and Older Adults*. NHS England Publications Gateway Reference 05958. https://www.england.nhs.uk/publication/achieving-better-access-to-247-urgent-and-emergency-mental-health-care-part-2-implementing-the-evidence-based-treatment-pathway-for-urgent-and-emergency-liaison-mental-health-services-for/ (last accessed September 2024).

RCEM (Royal College of Emergency Medicine) (2022). *RCEM Acute Insight Series: Mental Health Emergency Care*. https://rcem.ac.uk/wp-content/uploads/2022/09/RCEM-Acute-Insight-Series-Mental-Health-Emergency-Care.pdf (last accessed September 2024).

Chapter 2

NICE (National Institute for Health and Care Excellence) (2015). *Violence and Aggression: Short-Term Management in Mental Health, Health and Community Settings. NICE Guideline NG10*. www.nice.org.uk/guidance/ng10 (last accessed September 2024).

RCPsych (Royal College of Psychiatrists) (2011). *Standards on the use of Section 136 of the Mental Health Act 1983 (England and Wales)*. College Report CR159. https://www.rcpsych.ac.uk/docs/default-source/improving-care/better-mh-policy/college-reports/college-report-cr159.pdf (last accessed December 2024).

Chapter 3

SSVMS (Sierra Sacramento Valley Medical Society). *Smart Medical Clearance*.smartmedicalclearance.org (last accessed September 2024).

Acute Psychiatric Emergencies: A Practical Approach, Second Edition.
Edited by Mark Buchanan and Damien Longson.
© 2025 John Wiley & Sons Ltd. Published 2025 by John Wiley & Sons Ltd.

Chapter 4

eMentalHealth.ca/Primary Care. *Mental Status Examination (MSE)*. https://primarycare.ementalhealth.ca/index.php?m=fpArticle&ID=26974 (last accessed September 2024).

Chapter 6

ALSG (Advance Life Support Group) (2010). *Acute Medical Emergencies: The Practical Approach*, 2nd edn. Wiley-Blackwell, Oxford.

House A (2019). *Understanding and Responding to Self-Harm*. The One Stop Guide: *Practical Advice for Anybody Affected by Self-harm*. Profile Books, London.

Mackway-Jones K, Marsden J and Windle J (eds) (2013). *Emergency Triage*: *Manchester Triage Group*, 3rd edn.

NHS England (2024). *Guidance on Implementing the National Partnership Agreement: Right Care, Right Person*. https://www.england.nhs.uk/long-read/guidance-on-implementing-the-national-partnership-agreement-right-care-right-person/ (last accessed January 2025).

NHS England Digital (2023). *Emergency Care Data Set (ECDS)*. https:// digital. nhs.uk/data-and-information/data-collections-and-data-sets/ data-sets/ emergency-care-data-set-ecds (last accessed September 2024).

NHS England Digital (2024). *Hospital Episode Statistics (HES)*. https://digital. nhs.uk/data-and-information/data-tools-and-services/data-services/ hospital-episode-statistics (last accessed September 2024).

NICE (National Institute for Health and Care Excellence) (2022). *Self-harm: Assessment, Management and Preventing Recurrence*. NICE Guideline NG225. https://www.nice.org.uk/guidance/ng225 (last accessed September 2024).

RCEM (Royal College of Emergency Medicine) (2024). *The Patient who Absconds*. Best Practice Guideline. https://rcem.ac.uk/wp-content/ uploads/2024/08/Best_Practice_Guideline_The_Patient_Who_Absconds_ v1.pdf (last accessed October 2024).

RCPsych (Royal College of Psychiatrists), RCN (Royal College of Nursing), RCEM (Royal College of Emergency Medicine) and RCP (Royal College of Physicians) (2020). *Side by Side: a UK-wide consensus statement on working together to help patients with mental health needs in acute hospitals*. https://www.rcpsych.ac.uk/docs/default-source/members/ faculties/liaison-psychiatry/liaison-sidebyside.pdf (last accessed October 2024).

Sinclair J and Hawton K (2007) Suicide and deliberate self-harm. In: Lloyd GG and Guthrie E (eds) *Handbook of Liaison Psychiatry*. Cambridge University Press, Cambridge, pp. 245–269.

Chapter 7

Olshaker JS, Browne B, Jerrard DA, Prendergast H, Stair TO (1997). Medical clearance and screening of psychiatric patients in the emergency department. *Academic Emergency Medicine* 4(2), 124–128.

RCPsych (Royal College of Psychiatrists), RCN (Royal College of Nursing), RCEM (Royal College of Emergency Medicine) and RCP (Royal College of Physicians) (2020). *Side by Side: a UK-wide consensus statement on working together to help patients with mental health needs in acute hospitals.* https://www.rcpsych.ac.uk/docs/default-source/members/faculties/liaison-psychiatry/liaison-sidebyside.pdf (last accessed October 2024).

Chapter 8

NICE (National Institute for Health and Care Excellence) (2022). *Self-harm: Assessment, Management and Preventing Recurrence.* NICE Guideline NG225. https://www.nice.org.uk/guidance/ng225 (last accessed September 2024).

NICE (National Institute for Health and Care Excellence) (2023). *Head Injury: Assessment and Early Management.* NICE Guideline NG232. https://www.nice.org.uk/guidance/ng232 (last accessed September 2024).

RCPsych (Royal College of Psychiatrists), RCN (Royal College of Nursing), RCEM (Royal College of Emergency Medicine) and RCP (Royal College of Physicians) (2020). *Side by Side: a UK-wide consensus statement on working together to help patients with mental health needs in acute hospitals.* https://www.rcpsych.ac.uk/docs/default-source/members/faculties/liaison-psychiatry/liaison-sidebyside.pdf (last accessed October 2024).

Chapter 9

APA (American Psychiatric Association) (2013). *Diagnostic and Statistical Manual of Mental Disorders*, 5th edn. American Psychiatric Publishing,

WHO (World Health Organization) (2022). *International Classification of Diseases*, 11th edn. WHO, Geneva.

Chapter 10

Appelbaum PS, Robbins P and Monahan J (2000). Violence and delusions: data from the MacArthur Violence Risk Assessment Study. *American Journal of Psychiatry* 157(4), 566–572.

Baile WF, Buckman R, Lenzi R, et al. (2000) SPIKES – a six-step protocol for delivering bad news: application to the patient with cancer. *Oncologist* 5(4), 302–11.

Bjørkly S (1995). Prediction of aggression in psychiatric patients: a review of prospective prediction studies. *Clinical Psychology Review* 15(6), 475–502.

Castro M, Butler M, Thompson AN, Gee S and Posporelis S (2024). Effectiveness and safety of intravenous medications for the management of acute disturbance (agitation and other escalating behaviors): a systematic review of prospective interventional studies. *Journal of the Academy of Consultation-Liaison Psychiatry.* 65, 271–286.

Cowen P, Harrison P and Burns T (2012). *Shorter Oxford Textbook of Psychiatry*, 6th edn. Oxford University Press, Oxford.

Crilly J, Chaboyer W and Creedy D (2004). Violence towards emergency department nurses by patients. *Accident and Emergency Nursing* 12(2), 67–73.

Duxbury J (2002). An evaluation of staff and patient views of and strategies employed to manage inpatient aggression and violence on one mental health unit: a pluralistic design. *Journal of Psychiatric and Mental Health Nursing* 9(3), 325–337.

Duxbury J and Whittington R (2005). Causes and management of patient aggression and violence: staff and patient perspectives. *Journal of Advanced Nursing* 50(5), 469–478.

Elbogen EB and Johnson SC (2009). The intricate link between violence and mental disorder. *Archives of General Psychiatry* 66(2), 152.

Fluttert FAJ,Van Miejel B, Van Leeuwen M *et al.* (2011). The development of the forensic early warning signs of aggression Inventory: preliminary findings. *Archives of Psychiatric Nursing* 25(2), 129–137.

Foley S (2005). Incidence and clinical correlates of aggression and violence at presentation in patients with first episode psychosis. *Schizophrenia Research* 72(2/3), 161–168.

Gertz B (1980). Training for prevention of assaultive behavior in a psychiatric setting. *Psychiatric Services* 31(9), 628–630.

GMC (General Medical Council) (2018). *Confidentiality: Good Practice in Handling Patient Information*. https://www.gmc-uk.org/professional-standards/professional-standards-for-doctors/confidentiality (last accessed October 2024).

Gutierres SE and Van Puymbroeck C (2006). Childhood and adult violence in the lives of women who misuse substances. *Aggression and Violent Behavior* 11(5), 497–513.

Harrington JA (1972). Hospital violence (part 1). *Nursing Mirror* 135(4), 32–33.

Harris A and Lurigio AJ (2007). Mental illness and violence: a brief review of research and assessment strategies. *Aggression and Violent Behavior* 12(5), 542–551.

Jennings WG, Park M, Tomsich EA, Gover AR and Akers RL (2011). Assessing the overlap in dating violence perpetration and victimization among South Korean college students: the influence of social learning and self-control. *American Journal of Criminal Justice* 36(2), 188–206.

Johnson KL, Desmarais SL, Van Dorn RA and Grimm KJ (2014). A typology of community violence perpetration and victimization among adults with mental illnesses. *Journal of Interpersonal Violence* 30(3), 522–540.

Khwaja M and Beer MD (eds) (2012). *Prevention and Management of Violence: Guidance for Mental Healthcare Professionals*. College Report CR177. RCPsych Publications, Cambridge University Press, Cambridge.

Lavoie FW, Carter GL, Danzl DF and Berg RL (1988). Emergency department violence in United States teaching hospitals. *Annals of Emergency Medicine* 17(11), 1227–1233.

Lurigio AJ and Harris AJ (2009).Mental illness, violence, and risk assessment: an evidence-based review. *Victims and Offenders* 4(4), 341–347.

May DD and Grubbs LM (2002). The extent, nature, and precipitating factors of nurse assault among three groups of registered nurses in a Regional Medical Center. *Journal of Emergency Nursing* 28(1), 11–17.

McAllister R and Patel S (2012). Risk assessment and management. In: Khwaja M and Beer MD (eds) *Prevention and Management of Violence: Guidance for Mental Healthcare Professionals*. College Report CR177. RCPsych Publications, Cambridge University Press, Cambridge, pp. 13–17.

Monahan JT (2008). MacArthur Violence Risk Assessment Study. In: Butler BL (ed.) *Encyclopedia of Psychology and Law*. Sage, pp. 467–470.

Nijman HL (2002). A model of aggression in psychiatric hospitals. *Acta Psychiatrica Scandinavica* 106(S412), 142–143.

Nijman HL, aCampo JM, Ravelli DP and Merckelbach HL (1999). A tentative model of aggression on inpatient psychiatric wards. *Pyschiatric Services* 50(6), 832–834.

Pfeiffer C, Madray H, Ardolino A and Willms J (1998). The rise and fall of students' skill in obtaining a medical history. *Medical Education* 32(3), 283–288.

Pickard H and Fazel S (2013). Substance abuse as a risk factor for violence in mental illness. *Current Opinion in Psychiatry* 26(4), 349–354.

Price O and Baker J (2012). Key components of de-escalation techniques: a thematic synthesis. *International Journal of Mental Health Nursing* 21(4), 310–319.

Ramzi ZS, Fatah PW and Dalvandi A (2022). Prevalence of workplace violence against healthcare workers during the COVID-19 pandemic: a systematic review and meta-analysis. *Frontiers in Psychology* 13, 896156.

RCPsych (Royal College of Psychiatrists) (2017). *Assessment and Management of Risk to Others*. Good Practice Guide. https://www.rcpsych. ac.uk/docs/default-source/members/supporting-you/managing-and-assessing-risk/assessmentandmanagementrisktoothers.pdf (last accessed October 2024).

RCPsych (Royal College of Psychiatrists) (2023). *Assessing Risk: General Principles*. https://www.rcpsych.ac.uk/members/supporting-your-professional-development/assessing-and-managing-risk-of-patients-causing-harm/assessing-risk (last accessed September 2024).

Richmond JS, Berlin JS, Fishkind AB *et al.* (2012). Verbal de-escalation of the agitated patient: consensus statement of the American Association for Emergency Psychiatry Project BETA De-escalation Workgroup. *Western Journal of Emergency Medicine* 13(1), 17–25.

Rosell DR and Siever LJ (2015). The neurobiology of aggression and violence. *CNS Spectrums* 20(3), 254–279.

Siever LJ (2008). Neurobiology of aggression and violence. *American Journal of Psychiatry* 165(4), 429–442.

Soyka M (2000). Substance misuse, psychiatric disorder and violent and disturbed behaviour. *British Journal of Psychiatry* 176(4), 345–350.

Spidel A, Lecomte T, Greaves C, Sahlstrom K and Yuille JC (2010). Early psychosis and aggression: predictors and prevalence of violent behaviour amongst individuals with early onset psychosis. *International Journal of Law and Psychiatry* 33(3), 171–176.

Tiesman HM, Hendricks SA, Wiegand DM *et al.* (2023). Workplace violence and the mental health of public health workers during COVID-19. *American Journal of Preventive Medicine* 64(3), 315–325.

Ullrich S, Keers R and Coid JW (2013.) Delusions, anger, and serious violence: new findings from the MacArthur Violence Risk Assessment Study. *Schizophrenia Bulletin* 40(5), 1174–1181.

Whittington R and Wykes T (1994). An observational study of associations between nurse behaviour and violence in psychiatric hospitals. *Journal of Psychiatric and Mental Health Nursing* 1(2), 85–92.

Yap CYL, Daniel C, Knott JC, Myers E and Gerdtz M (2023). Causes and management of aggression and violence: a survey of emergency department nurses and attendees. *International Emergency Nursing* 69, 101292.

Chapter 11

MBRRACE-UK (2023). *Saving Lives, Improving Mothers' Care. State of the Nation Surveillance Report: Surveillance Findings from the UK Confidential Enquiries into Maternal Deaths 2019–21.* National Perinatal Epidemiology Unit, University of Oxford, Oxford.

RCPsych (Royal College of Psychiatrists) (2022). *Medical Emergencies in Eating Disorders: Guidance on Recognition and Management.* College Report CR233. https://www.rcpsych.ac.uk/improving-care/campaigning-for-better-mental-health-policy/college-reports/2022-college-reports/cr233 (last accessed October 2024).

Chapter 12

HCPC (Health and Care Professionals Council) (2020). *Guidance on Confidentiality.* https://www.hcpc-uk.org/standards/meeting-our-standards/confidentiality/guidance-on-confidentiality/ (last accessed October 2024).

Chapter 13

Flin R, O'Connor P and Crichton M (2008). *Safety at the Sharp End: A Guide to Non-technical Skills.* CRC Press, Aldershot.

Tversky A and Kahneman D (1974). Judgment under uncertainty: heuristics and biases. *Science* 185(4157), 1124–1131.

Index

Page references in *italics* refer to figures

Acute Psychiatric Emergencies: A Practical Approach, Second Edition.
Edited by Mark Buchanan and Damien Longson.
© 2025 John Wiley & Sons Ltd. Published 2025 by John Wiley & Sons Ltd.